Reviews and critical articles covering the entire field of normal anatomy (cytology, histology, cyto- and histochemistry, electron microscopy, macroscopy, experimental morphology and embryology and comparative anatomy) are published in Advances in Anatomy, Embryology and Cell Biology. Papers dealing with anthropology and clinical morphology that aim to encourage co-operation between anatomy and related disciplines will also be accepted. Papers are normally commissioned. Original papers and communications may be submitted and will be considered for publication provided they meet the requirements of a review article and thus fit into the scope of "Advances". English language is preferred, but in exceptional cases French or German papers will be accepted.

It is a fundamental condition that submitted manuscripts have not been and will not simultaneously be submitted or published elsewhere. With the acceptance of a manuscript for publication, the publisher acquires full and exclusive copyright for all languages and countries.

Twenty-five copies of each paper are supplied free of charge.

Manuscripts should be addressed to

Prof. Dr. F. **BECK,** Howard Florey Institute, University of Melbourne, Parkville, 3000 Melbourne, Victoria, Australia

Prof. Dr. B. **CHRIST**, Anatomisches Institut der Universität Freiburg, Abteilung Anatomie II, Albertstr. 17, D-79104 Freiburg, Germany

Prof. Dr. W. **KRIZ,** Anatomisches Institut der Universität Heidelberg, Im Neuenheimer Feld 307, D-69120 Heidelberg, Germany

Prof. Dr. W. **KUMMER**, Institut für Anatomie und Zellbiologie, Universität Gießen, Aulweg 123, D-35385 Gießen, Germany

Prof. Dr. E. **MARANI**, Leiden University, Department of Physiology, Neuroregulation Group, P.O. Box 9604, 2300 RC Leiden, The Netherlands

Prof. Dr. R. **PUTZ**, Anatomische Anstalt der Universität München, Lehrstuhl Anatomie I, Pettenkoferstr. 11, D-80336 München, Germany

Prof. Dr. Dr. h.c. Y. **SANO,** Department of Anatomy, Kyoto Prefectural University of Medicine, Kawaramachi-Hirokoji, 602 Kyoto, Japan

Prof. Dr. Dr. h.c. T. H. **SCHIEBLER,** Anatomisches Institut der Universität, Koellikerstraße 6, D-97070 Würzburg, Germany

Ph. D. Gary C. **SCHOENWOLF,** Department of Neurobiology and Anatomy, University of Utah School of Medicine, 50 N. Medical Drive, Salt Lake City, Utah 84132, USA

Prof. Dr. K. **ZILLES**, Universität Düsseldorf, Medizinische Einrichtungen, C. u. O. Vogt-Institut, Postfach 101007, D-40001 Düsseldorf, Germany

Advances in Anatomy
Embryology and Cell Biology

Vol. 168

Springer-Verlag Berlin Heidelberg GmbH

M. von Lüdinghausen

The Venous Drainage of the Human Myocardium

With 35 Figures and 12 Tables

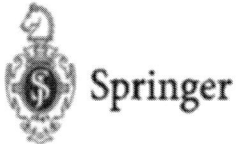 Springer

Prof. Dr. Michael von Lüdinghausen

Institut für Anatomie und Zellbiologie,
Universität Würzburg,
Koellikerstr. 6,
97070 Würzburg, Germany
e-mail: anat033@mail.uni-wuerzburg.deauthorinfo

ISSN 0301-5556
ISBN 978-3-540-44017-8

Library of Congress-Cataloging-in-Publication-Data
The Clinical Anatomy of Coronary Arteries / M. v. Lüdinghausen – Berlin;
Heidelberg; New York: Springer, 2003
   (Advances in anatomy, embryology, and cell biology; Vol. 168)
   ISBN 978-3-540-44017-8   ISBN 978-3-642-55623-4 (eBook)
   DOI 10.1007/978-3-642-55623-4

http://www.springer.de

© Springer-Verlag Berlin Heidelberg 2003
Originally published by Springer-Verlag Berlin Heidelberg New York in 2003

Production: PRO EDIT GmbH, 69126 Heidelberg, Germany
Printed on acid-free paper   27/3150Re – 5 4 3 2 1 0

Contents

1 Introduction

Enhanced performance, evaluation, and interpretation of the various forms of cardiological diagnostic procedures and open-heart surgery, the achievement of a rapid improvement in the oxygen consumption of hypoxic myocardium, and the salvage of viable but ischemic myocardium still appear to constitute the most important challenges to modern medicine.

Research on the vascular anatomy of the myocardium has mostly been focused on the coronary arteries and myocardial capillaries (von Lüdinghausen 2002); by comparison, the coronary or cardiac venous systems have traditionally been neglected. A search through the literature of the mid-twentieth century onwards fails to reveal a detailed report on the anatomy and topography of the coronary sinus (CS) and its related veins (Smith 1962).

In this area, new frontiers have been crossed through the use of the technique of CS catheterization, for instance for the purpose of:

1. The visualization of the venous part of cardiac circulation [angiography, computed tomography (CT)]. Methods of visualization of the coronary venous drainage system using electron-beam CT and angiographical methods have recently been presented by Schaffler et al. (2000) and Sun et al. (2002).
2. Electro-physiological study of the atrial components of the conduction system. The morphology of accessory pathways of the conduction system in the neighborhood of the CS, their diagnostics and surgical treatment have been investigated and discussed by Becker et al. (1978), Seally and Mikat (1983), Robinson et al. (1988), and Sun et al. (2002).
3. The venous reperfusion of the ventricular myocardium. During the past 50 years, enormous advances have been made in augmenting blood flow to the ischemic myocardium. Many clinicians have great optimism where the method of CS catheterization and venous reperfusion is concerned; the reasons for this are presented briefly here (Mohl et al. 1992).

1.1
Goal of CS Catheterization

The reperfusion technique permits the protection of underperfused myocardium by catheterization of the CS and perfusion of its related veins (Pratt 1898; Beck 1948; Beck and Leighninger 1954; Sallam and Kolff 1973; Menasche et al. 1982; Mohl 1984a, 2000; Jacobs 1986; Lazar 1988) and enables a reverse nourishment of the myocardium, which is otherwise – for instance during lengthy open-heart surgery with induced cardiac arrest or in a case of obstructive coronary atherosclerosis – threatened by ischemia and infarction. The physiologist Pratt (1898) was the first to publish the technique and its results after performing animal experiments, but these have almost been forgotten. Fifty years later, Beck et al. (1948) rediscovered this simple but brilliant idea and recommended it for clinical application.

Since then, cardiologists and heart surgeons have sought more and detailed information of the anatomical organization, distribution patterns, topographical relationships, and variable modes of opening of the CS and the different types of cardiac veins (Arom and Emery 1992).

1.2
Objective of the Study

The objective of this study is to present comprehensive morphological data, a considerable amount new, about the venous drainage of the human myocardium. This information is not only of great significance for the successful performance of CS catheterization and evaluation of myocardial reperfusion but also for the angiographic presentation and evaluation of the distribution pattern and function of cardiac veins.

2 The Organization of the Cardiac Venous Systems

Transverse sections through the walls of the left ventricle and the interventricular septum have shown three zones of venous vascularization:
1. The external epicardial zone comprising a thin, external layer (about 1 mm in thickness) of the free walls of the left ventricle
2. The medial subepicardial (thickest) zone, which together with the external zone constitutes about two-thirds of the total thickness of the walls of the left ventricle and adjacent IV septum
3. The internal subendocardial zone, comprising the remainder of the walls of the left ventricle and IV septum facing this ventricle (Pakalska and Golab 1980)

In the walls of the right ventricle only two zones of venous vascularization were observed:
1. The external epicardial zone comprising about 1 mm thickness of the external layer of the walls of the right ventricle) (Figs.1, 2)
2. The internal zone comprising the whole thickness (equal to that of both the medial subepicardial and the internal subendocardial zones) of the wall of the right ventricle, in contrast to the internal zone of the wall of the left ventricle as mentioned above (Figs. 1, 2)

On the basis of the findings from research carried out by anatomists, physiologists, and cardiologists, the system of cardiac circulation has been divided into three parts:
1. The greater or major cardiac venous system (GCVS) (Figs. 1, 2)
2. The smaller or minor cardiac venous system (SCVS) (Bohning et al. 1933; Wearn et al. 1933; Lindenau and Romaniuk 1983; Mohl 1984b) (Figs. 1, 2)
3. The compound system consisting of a) intramyocardial sinusoids and b) intramyocardial sinuses and tunnels which exhibit morphological details of both the GCVS and the SCVS (Figs. 1, 2)

According to Pakalska and Golab (1980) and Lametschwandtner et al. (1990), the venous filling of all zones of the walls of the ventricles is dependent upon the pressure used to inject the veins under examination. A pressure below 50 mm Hg filled only the veins of the external and medial zones, whereas pressures of up to 80 mm Hg filled the veins in all the myocardial zones of the ventricular walls.

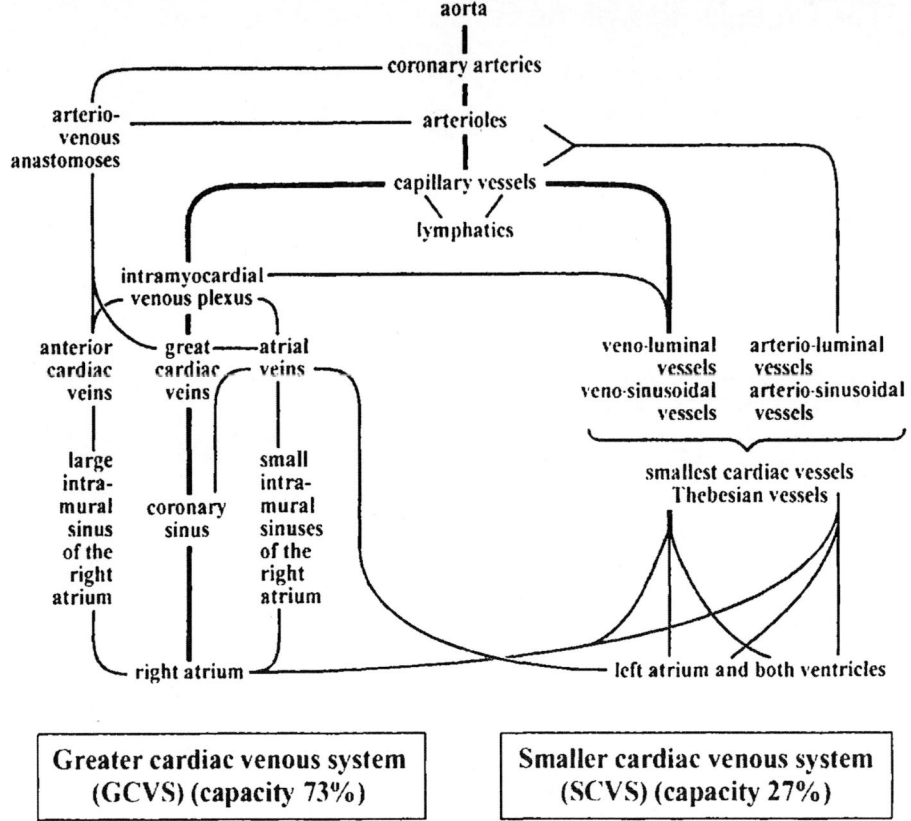

Fig. 1. Schematic drawing to illustrate the distribution pattern and interconnections of the tributaries of the greater (*GCVS*) and smaller cardiac vascular systems (*SCVS*)

2.1
The Greater (Major) Cardiac Venous System

Definition. The vessels of the GCVS are located within the subepicardial layer which extends over the surface of the ventricular and atrial myocardium. It is noticeable that the veins of the GCVS often ignore topographical borders such as those presented by the coronary, interventricular and interatrial sulci, or even leave the heart by crossing the porta venosa, and that they exhibit relatively large ostial valves (von Lüdinghausen et al. 1995) (Figs. 1, 2).

Classification. The GCVS consists of several intercommunicating parts:
1. The CS and its ventricular tributaries
2. The anterior cardiac venous system
3. The superior veins of the interventricular septum
4. The left atrial veins
5. The mediastinal tributaries to both atria
6. The right atrial veins

4

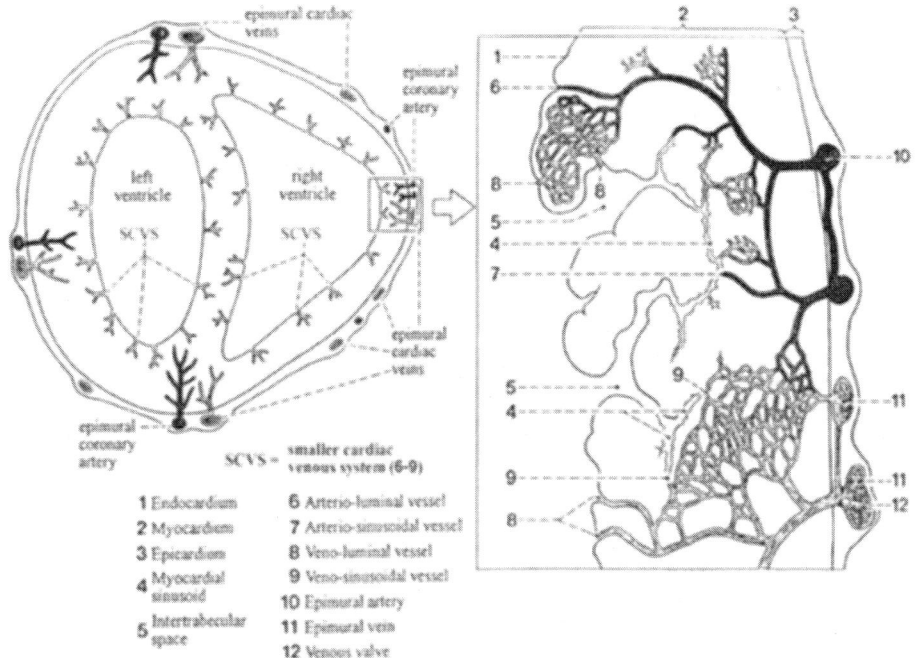

Fig. 2. Distribution pattern of the cardiac vessels in the myocardium of the ventricular walls. *Left:* Schematic drawing of a cross-section through the ventricles showing the vessels of the GCVS on the myocardial surface and those of the SCVS in the subendocardial layers. *Right:* Enlargement of a section of the left ventricle (indicated by a *rectangle*) showing the arrangement of the epimurally distributed coronary arteries and cardiac veins, the intramural distribution of their branches, and their relation to subendocardial vessels

Development of the Coronary Sinus. Developmentally, the CS is a remnant of the left horn of the sinus venosus and is, therefore, part of the right atrium (Goerttler 1963; Langman 1977; Moore 1988; Tschabitscher 1984; Steding et al. 1990).

After incorporation of the sinus venosus into the right atrium, the sinus septum participates in the subdivision of the right sinus valve into the ostial valves of both the CS and inferior vena cava (according to Yater 1929; Steding et al. 1990).

The oblique vein of the left atrium has its origin in the proximal part of the left cardinal vein in the embryo (Netter 1976).

Remnants of the right valve of the embryonic sinus venosus are not uncommon and are recognized as the normal ostial valves of the CS and inferior vena cava. Trento et al. (1988) found a few cases of prominent ostial valves which divided the right atrium into two parts.

2.2
The Smaller (Minor) Cardiac Venous System

Definition. In mammalian hearts, there are multiple small and thin direct vascular communications between the coronary arteries and the chambers of the heart consisting of channels, lacunae, and sinusoids in the subendocardial layers of the atrial and ventricular walls. These have been collectively named smallest cardiac vessels; the majority of them together constitute the *smaller cardiac venous system* (Wearn 1928; Grant and Viko 1929; Wearn et al. 1933; Unger 1938; Hammond and Austen 1967; Heine 1976).

Numerous minute orifices of the vessels of the SCVS are found in particular in the septal and right lateral walls of the right and (though less often) the left atrium (Pratt 1898; Spalteholz 1934; Esperanca Pina and Dos Santos Ferreira 1974; Esperanca Pina and Trindade 1977; Tschabitscher 1984; Lechleuthner and von Lüdinghausen 1986; Rosinia and Low 1986; Waller and Schlant 1994). Ostia of smallest cardiac vessels are also frequently found on the surface of papillary muscles.

It is generally accepted that the vessels of the SCVS connect not only the intramural coronary system and the chambers of the heart but also prevent retroflow and eventual myocardial nourishment (Pratt 1898; Bohning et al. 1933; Lendrum et al. 1945; Gould 1953; Friedell 1966; Heintzberger 1984; Lindenau and Romaniuk 1983; Rosinia and Low 1986).

Vajda et al. (1972) determined and measured connections between subepicardially distributed veins and the lymphatics of the human heart (Figs. 1).

Classification. The vessels of the SCVS comprise the following four types (Wearn 1928; Grant and Viko 1929; Wearn et al. 1933; Prinzmetal et al. 1947; Gould 1953; Baroldi and Scomazzoni 1965; Schaper 1974; Lindenau and Romaniuk 1983; Lunkenheimer et al. 1984; Heintzberger 1984; Moscovici 1985; Lametschwandtner and Mohl 1984; Ratajczyk-Pakalska and Kolff 1984; Tschabitscher 1984; Ansari 2001):

1. Veno-sinusoidal vessels, which as the smallest veins (venules) connect intramural veins with subendocardial sinusoids and drain the internal layers of the atrial and ventricular myocardium
2. Veno-luminal vessels, which connect intramural venous networks with the atria or ventricles
3. Arterio-sinusoidal vessels which connect thin arteries or arterioles with sinusoidal spaces in the internal walls of the atria or ventricles
4. Arterio-luminal vessels which connect small arteries or arterioles with atria or ventricles

Distribution. With the use of injected adult human heart specimens for microanatomical and histological investigations (Nerantzis et al. 1978; Pakalska and Golab 1980; Ratajczyk-Pakalska and Kolff 1984; Ansari 2001) and through the study of corrosion casts of human heart specimens by scanning electron microscopy (SEM) (Lametschwandtner and Mohl 1984; Tschabitscher 1984; Ono et al. 1986; Lechleuthner 1987; von Lüdinghausen et al. 1995), it is possible to visualize the smallest vessels in the subendocardial layers. These tenuous vessels are highly variable in form (arboriform, sinuous, canal-like) size, number, and length (on average about 15 mm); they run in all directions, obviously without orientation, are interconnected with larger veins of the medial zone (Grant and Viko 1929; Bohning et al. 1933; Ratajczyk-Pakalska and Kolff 1984; Ansari 2001), and have tiny outlets draining the subendocardial myocardium directly into the cardiac chambers, most frequently the right atrium (RA) and right ventricle (RV). They are more absent in the left heart chambers (Aho 1950). The very short vessels have an ostial diameter of less than 0.5 mm (Waller and

Schlant 1994). Most of the openings are not visible to the naked eye in a cadaver specimen.

Histology. From the histological point of view, the vessels of the SCVS do not have a proper muscular wall. According to Robb (1965), the endothelial linings of the vessels of the SCVS continue the endothelium of the heart cavities.

SEM of Mercox-injected casts revealed a clearer branching pattern of the smallest subendocardial and intramyocardial vessels in heart specimens from various species of animals (Phillips et al. 1979; Anderson and Anderson 1981; Lametschwandtner and Mohl 1984; Lechleuthner 1987). These veins almost always lack an effective protective or occlusive valve leaflet at their openings; instead, the ventricular or atrial endocardial openings may exhibit simple endothelial folds or sphincters of a few smooth muscle cells (Pakalska et al. 1981; Ratajczyk-Pakalska et al. 1984; Ratajczyk-Pakalska and Kolff 1984; Lechleuthner and von Lüdinghausen 1986).

The smallest cardiac vessels and cardiac sinusoids are capable of collecting large quantities of venous blood (Schlant and Sonnenblick 1994) and bringing sufficient nutriment from the ventricular cavities to the myocardium in order to maintain rhythmic contractions for a continuous and long period of time. Their capacity is about 27%, which includes 22% accounted for by the smallest cardiac vessels. The capacity of the arterio-luminal and arterio-sinusoidal vessels alone is about 5% (Hammond and Austen 1967; Hochberg and Austen 1980).

Cardiac Sinusoids (Sinusoidal Channels or Outpocketings). As is the case with sinusoids in other organs, the cardiac sinusoids are similar to capillaries in that they have a simple wall of endothelium and a few loose connective tissue fibers. They differ from capillaries in having a lumen whose diameter and contour varies over its whole length. In some areas, a sinusoid may have expanded into a spacious vessel many times the diameter of a capillary (30–200 μm in diameter according to Roberts 1958), while in others, the sinusoid may be constricted in an irregular way with some protrusion of endothelial cells into the lumen.

The richly anastomosing network of thin-walled irregular sinusoids in all ventricular walls has been well described by Voboril and Schiebler (1970), Rychter and Ostadal (1971), Lunkenheimer and Merker (1973), Lunkenheimer et al. (1984), Heintzberger (1984), and Moscovici (1985). The sinusoids receive vessels from the intramyocardial arterioles, the capillary bed, and the cardiac venules, and they empty – passing intertrabecular spaces – directly into the lumen of the heart. The sinusoids are lined with a single layer of endothelium and range from 40 to 75 μm in diameter in dogs, and 60 to 90 μm in the septal myocardium of the newborn human (Gregg and Fisher 1963).

Clinical Remark. The myocardial sinusoids, to which the previously-used terms "arterio-sinusoidal" and "veno-sinusoidal" vessels refer, may be regarded as intertrabecular spaces of much-reduced caliber.

These tiny vessels and the previously discussed arterio-luminal and veno-luminal vessels enable a direct short-cut between the smallest coronary arteries and cardiac veins and the four heart chambers, and are part of the original Thebesian veins (Bohning et al. 1933).

The latter-mentioned two categories of vessels are also termed physiological arterio-venous anastomoses (Ratajczyk-Pakalska 1977).

Persistent communicating intertrabecular sinusoidal spaces of embryological origin in adult myocardium may develop pathological arterio-luminal or arterio-myocardial fistulae, which may be associated with coronary artery steal syndrome and angina pectoris. (Singer et al. 1973; Theman and Crosby 1981).

On the other hand, discussion has centered around the ability of the vessels of the SCVS to enable a reverse blood flow from the ventricles into the inner layers of the ventricular myocardium in cases of diminished arterial supply.

The complex issue of myocardial microcirculation is not discussed further in this work.

History. For almost 200 years the vessels of the SCVS have synonymously and collectively been named Thebesian veins (Thebesius 1708; Bochdalek 1868; Pratt 1898; Wearn 1928; Gregg and Dewald 1938; Aho 1950; Bargmann 1963), although Vieussens (1706) found and described them independently, at an earlier date than Thebesius. It was the discovery made by Vieussens (1706) and Thebesius (1708) which showed that small cardiac vessels directly conduct blood from peripheral areas of the cardiac walls, i.e., from the coronary system, into the heart chambers. This has subsequently been confirmed by many researchers (Abernethy 1798; Langer 1880; Wearn 1928; Grant and Viko 1929; Spalteholz 1934; Mettenleiter 2001). They have also been designated as "fleshy ducts" or "lacunae," and "ductus," "ductuli carnosi," or just Thebesian veins (Bochdalek 1868; Baroldi and Scomazzoni 1965; Rosinia and Low 1986).

Bochdalek (1868), Langer (1880), Wearn (1928), Wearn et al. (1933), and Gregg and Dewald (1938) repeated the experiments of Vieussens and Thebesius (ligation of the CS and study of alternative drainage routes for cardiac venous blood or colored dye) and confirmed the results. According to the original manuscript of Thebesius (1708), the anterior cardiac veins (ACVs) were parts of the alternative venous drainage routes.

At the end of the nineteenth century, the ACVs were accepted as constituting a separate group of large non-coronary veins (Bochdalek 1868; Langer 1880).

Subsequently, all tiny cardiac veins were named *smallest cardiac veins* or vv cardiacae cordis minimae, when they did not terminate in the CS and did not belong amongst the ACVs, and when they had their own small openings (almost invisible to the naked eye) on the endocardial surface of the right and left cardiac chambers (Wearn et al. 1933; Bargmann 1963; Baroldi and Scomazzoni 1965; Singer et al. 1973; McAlpine 1975; Vlodaver et al. 1976; Fleischhauer 1985; Frick et al. 1987; Leonhard 1987; Williams et al. 1995; Feneis and Dauber 1998).

Smallest Cardiac Veins or Smallest Cardiac Vessels? Even though the all-inclusive term Thebesian veins has hitherto been used, it should no longer be applied because it is not of a sufficiently exact and precise nature to describe the variable and complex characters of these vessels (Mettenleiter 2001). In view of their arterial components, it is more consistent and appropriate to change the designations of "smallest cardiac veins" or "Thebesian veins" to "smallest cardiac vessels" or "Thebesian vessels" (Bohning et al. 1933; Grant 1926; Grant and Viko 1929; Esperanca Pina and Trindade 1977; Pakalska and Golab 1980; Pakalska et al. 1981; von Lüdinghausen 1987).

Development of the Smallest Cardiac Vessels. Investigation of the embryology of the smallest cardiac vessels in mammalian hearts has indicated that they represent the remains of the primitive cardiac circulation (Voboril and Schiebler 1969; Steding and Seidl 1980); the latter effects the supply and drainage of the spongeous intertrabecular myocardium of the developing heart, usually to the next adjacent chamber (Lunken-heimer et al. 1984; Tschabitscher 1984; Moore 1988). The embryonic sinusoidal circulation is more than sufficient to nourish the trabeculae. In the adult heart, a few of the sinusoids of embryological origin survive as intertrabecular spaces; these constitute the smallest cardiac vessels (Wearn 1928; Gould 1953; O'Rahilly 1971; Dusek et al. 1975; Steding and Seidl 1980; Moore 1988; Christ 1990).

According to Robb (1965), the endothelial linings of the smallest cardiac vessels derive from the endothelium of the heart cavities. Therefore, these vessels may be called phylogenetic remnants of the extensive sinusoidal blood supply coursing from the heart chambers in the embryo. They are found not only in mammalian hearts, but also in the hearts of fully-grown fish and reptiles (Lewis 1904; Grant and Regnier 1926; Lunkenheimer and Merker 1974).

2.3
The Compound Form of Cardiac Venous Vessels:
Intramural Sinuses and Tunnels

In the walls of both atria there are frequently occurring, variably-sized (small or large, short or long) subendocardial and intramural sinuses and tunnels of 3–70 mm length and 2–5 mm width. Each of these exhibits characteristics of both the GCVS and SCVS. Thus, they constitute either enlarged spaces of the SCVS or intramurally integrated terminal parts of veins belonging to the GCVS.

These sinuses and tunnels have frequently been found situated in, and attached to, the external walls of the right atrium and the interatrial septum. These vascular spaces collect blood either from the left atrial veins or from the anterior cardiac veins (Mochizuki 1933; Parsonnet 1953; Tschabitscher 1984; von Lüdinghausen et al. 1984; Ortale and Marquez 1998).

3 Nomenclature

In this work, the accepted terminology of the coronary sinus and its tributaries is used in its English and Latin versions according to Nomina Anatomica (1980, 1989, 1998), von Lüdinghausen et al. (1984), and Terminologia Anatomica (1998).

3.1
English and Latin Versions

The English names are given in italics and the Latin names in parentheses:
- *Superior vena cava* (v cava superior)
- *Inferior vena cava* (v cava inferior)
- *Ostial valve of the inferior vena cava* (Valva ostii venae cavae inferioris)
- *Coronary sinus* (Sinus coronarius)
- *Ostial angle of the coronary sinus* (Angulus ostii sinus coronarii)
- *Ostial valve of the coronary sinus* (Valvula ostii sinus coronarii)
- *Coronary sulcus or atrioventricular sulcus* (Sulcus coronarius or Sulcus atrioventricularis)
- *Great cardiac vein or left coronary vein* (v cardiaca magna or v coronaria sinistra), consisting of two parts: the *anterior interventricular vein* and its continuation, the *left coronary vein*
- *Ostial valve of the great cardiac vein* (Valvula ostii venae cardiacae magnae)
- *Anterior interventricular vein* (v interventricularis anterior)
- *Left marginal vein* (v marginalis sinistra)
- *Posterior vein of the left ventricle, posterior left ventricular vein* (v posterior ventriculi sinistri)
- *Posterior interventricular vein* (v interventricularis posterior)
- *Small cardiac vein or right coronary vein* (v cardiaca parva or v coronaria dextra)
- *Right marginal vein* (v marginalis dextra)
- *Anterior cardiac veins* (vv cardiacae anteriores)
- *Oblique vein of the left atrium* (v obliqua atrii sinistri)
- *Conus vein(s)* [v(v) coni arteriosi]
- *Smallest cardiac veins/vessels* (vv cardiacae minimae or vv cordis minimae)

3.2
Abbreviations

ACVs	Anterior cardiac veins
AIV	Anterior interventricular vein
AO	Aorta
AOCS	Atrial ostium of the coronary sinus
AVs	Atrial veins
CS	Coronary sinus
IVC	Inferior vena cava
IV sulcus, septum	Interventricular sulcus, septum
IV artery, branch	Interventricular artery, branch
GCVS	Greater cardiac venous system
GCV	Great cardiac vein
LA	Left atrium
LMV	Left marginal vein
LSSV	Left superior septal vein
LV	Left ventricle
MI	Mitral valve
OV	Oblique vein of the left atrium; Marshalls vein
PIV	Posterior interventricular vein
PT	Pulmonary trunk
PVLV	Posterior vein of the left ventricle
PVs	Pulmonary veins
RA	Right atrium
RMV	Right marginal vein
RSSV	Right superior septal vein
RV	Right ventricle
SA node	Sinuatrial node
SCVS	Smaller cardiac venous system
SCV	Small cardiac vein
SVs	Septal veins
SVC	Superior vena cava
TRI	Tricuspid valve
VT(s)RA	Venous tunnel(s) of the right atrium

3.3
Commonly Used Unofficial or Alternative Terms and Synonyms for the Cardiac Veins

In addition to the official nomenclature, there are some other older, but still commonly used, unofficial or alternative terms for the cardiac veins (in italics). The Latin terms are given in parentheses.
- *Inferior caval vein* (v cava inferior)
- *Superior caval vein* (v cava superior)
- *Middle cardiac vein* (v interventricularis posterior)
- *Eustachian valve* (Valva ostii venae cavae inferioris)

- *Thebesian valve* (Valvula ostii sinus coronarii)
- *Valve of Vieussens* (Valvula ostii venae cardiacae magnae)
- *Veins of Vieussens* (vv cardiacae anteriores including veins which drain the adipose tissue covering the conus arteriosus)
- *Vein of Cruveilhiers* (v coni arteriosi)
- *Vein of Zuckerkandl* (draining the soft tissue between the aortic root and the pulmonary trunk and emptying directly into the right atrium)
- *Galens vein* (v marginalis dextra)
- *Marshalls vein* (v obliqua atrii sinistri)
- Cuvieris duct (v cava superior sinistra persistens)
- *Thebesian veins or vessels, Thebesian foramina* (vv cardiacae minimae; foramina venarum cardiacarum minimarum)
- *Venous tunnel of the RA* (Mochizuki 1933), *intramural venous sinus of the RA, subendocardial vein of the RA* (Parsonnet 1953), *intramyocardial vein of the RA, common channel of the RA* (Esperanca Pina 1975), *right coronary collecting channel, venous lake of the RA* (McAlpine 1975), *collecting vein of the RA* (Waller and Schlant 1994), *right coronary sinus* (von Lüdinghausen and Schott 1990).
- *Waterston sulcus* (Sulcus interatrialis posterior)

4
Microanatomy of the Coronary Sinus

4.1
Anatomy, Position, and Topography

Anatomy. The CS is the most constant feature of the system of cardiac venous outflow. Although numerous variations in its position, shape, size, length, and diameter have been reported, it can be stated that, as a rule, in a man with a weight of 80 kg, the sinus is 40 mm in length and 10 mm in diameter (McAlpine 1975), that is to say, the CS is usually somewhat smaller than a human little finger (Figs. 3, 4).

Position and Topography. The CS is situated in the posterior portion of the coronary sulcus on the diaphragmatic (posterior) surface of the heart. It extends from the left ventricular margin and the opening of the OV to empty into the RA via an atrial orifice in the crux cordis area (McAlpine 1975; Anderson and Becker 1982; Williams et al. 1995; von Lüdinghausen and Schott 1990; Maric et al. 1996).

The CS receives most of the epicardial ventricular veins: the OV (and some other left and right atrial veins), the AIV and its continuation, the GCV, furthermore the PVLV, the LMV, and the PIV (Mochizuki 1933, Silver and Rowley 1988).

The arched course of the GCV continues in the CS, namely in the posterior part of the left coronary sulcus. Here it runs parallel to the circumflex branch of the left coronary artery and enters the posterior aspect of the RA (Vlodaver et al. 1976). The CS courses almost parallel to the attachment of the mural (posterior) leaflet of the MI.

The position of the CS in the left half of the posterior coronary sulcus is well known. It extends from the OV to the so-called crux cordis, which is the conjunction of the posterior IV sulcus and coronary sulcus. In the adult (as seen in cadaver specimens), the CS has a cylindrical or conal shape and is the size of the distal and middle phalanx of an adult little finger (Williams et al. 1995; Waller and Schlant 1994).

Although actually part of the right atrium, the CS is consistently seen with a myocardial wall or a surrounding myocardial coat on the postero-inferior wall of the left atrium (Langman 1977; Moore 1988) (Figs. 3, 4).

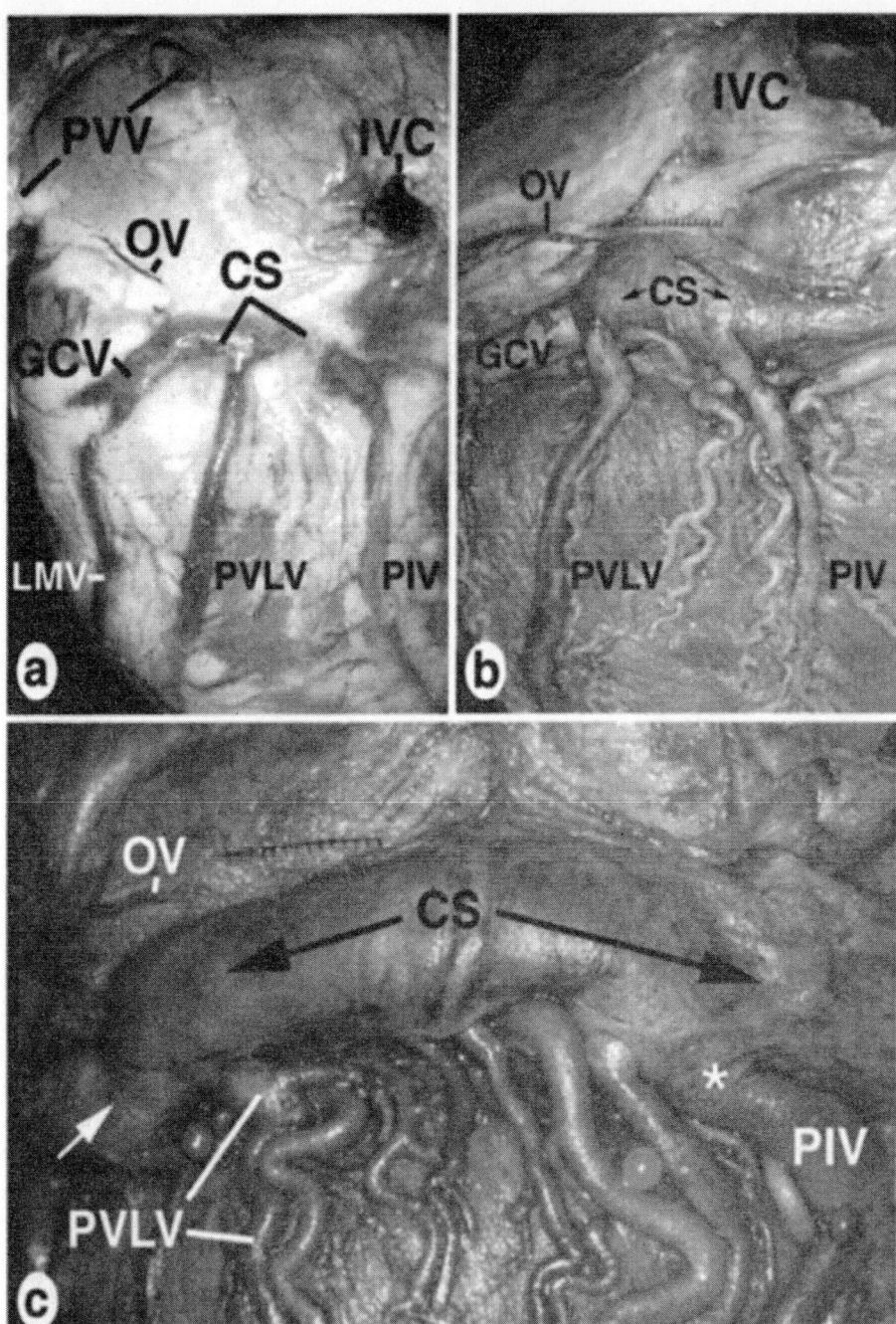

Fig. 3a–c. Diaphragmatic surface of human heart specimens. a The coronary sinus (*CS*) and its major tributaries are visible through the transparent visceral pericardium. b A rather short CS (exposed). c A rather long CS (exposed). In a and c the terminal part of the great cardiac vein (*GCV*) appears kinked as it leaves the coronary sulcus and continues into the CS; the terminal parts of both the GCV (*white arrow*) and PIV (indicated by a *white asterisk*) are wrapped within the myocardial coat of the CS

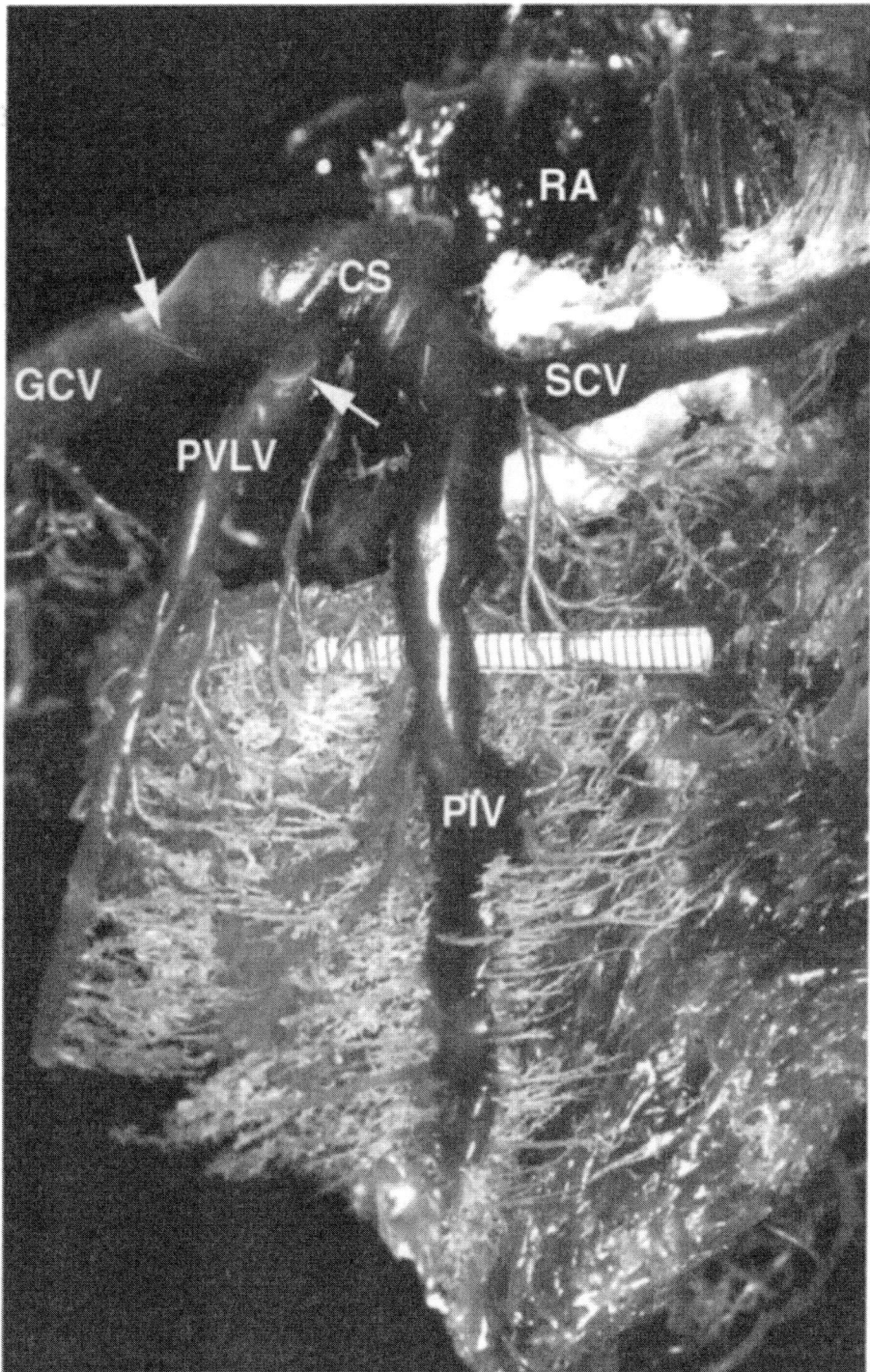

Fig. 4. Posterior surface of a corrosion cast of the CS and its major tributaries; the CS is quite short. A unicuspid ostial valve is visible in the terminal sections of both the GCV and the PVLV (marked by *white arrows*). No valve is visible in the terminal section of the PIV and the SCV

4.2
Surface Anatomy

The confluence of the GCV and the CS occurs at a point along the terminal section of the OV; the vein subsequently descends and runs along its posterior wall. In many cases the OV is translucent and visible through the epicardium; therefore, the beginning of the CS is clearly discernible (Bargmann 1963; Anderson and Becker 1982). The myocardial cover of the CS, because of its irregular extension, is not a suitable starting-point from which the confluence of the terminal part of the GCV and the initial part of the CS can be determined (von Lüdinghausen et al. 1992). Furthermore, it is impossible to determine the exact location of the atrial ostium of the CS on the external diaphragmatic surface of the heart, because there is no conspicuous landmark in the posterior coronary sulcus or in the area of the crux cordis which corresponds to the right atrial ostium or indicates its location within the depth of the crux (von Lüdinghausen and Schott 1990).

Roberts (1958) describes a prominent dimple or funnel-shaped depression in the angle just above the orifice of the CS and to the left of the end of the IVC. The author designates it a useful landmark for the determination of the atrial end of the CS (Fig. 3).

4.3
Length and Shape

After axial section of the CS, its length was measured between the entrance of the OV and the base of the ostial valve of the CS (Table 1). Both length and shape exhibited numerous variations in the cases examined. The length varied between 15 and 70 mm, but in 75% of the cases it lay between 30 and 50 mm (Table 2). In individuals who have had severe congestive heart failure, especially those with right atrial hypertension or with extensive hypertrophy of the heart, the diameter of the CS may be several times the normal average, with a widely patent atrial orifice. There was one case of cardiomegaly (790 g) in our material, in which the CS had an extreme length measuring 82 mm (Figs. 3, 4, 5a–c).

Table 1. Length of the CS (the averages of the measurements are given in parentheses)

Tandler (1926)	20–65 mm
Parsonnet (1953)	15–53 mm (35 mm)
Roberts (1958)	20–50 mm
Malhotra et al. (1980)	20–40 mm
Silver and Rowley (1988)	17–65 mm
Maric et al. (1996)	21–45 mm (33.9 mm)
Own material	15–70 mm (37.0 mm)

Table 2. Diameters, cross-sectional areas, circumferences, volumes of the CS (the averages of the measurements are given in parentheses)

Origin of CS, cross-sect. area	(Silver and Rowley 1988)	13–38 (20.6) mm^2
	(Silver and Rowley 1988)	13–79 (28) mm^{2*}
Midcoronary sinus, diameter	(Tandler 1926)	6–16 mm
	(Ortale et al. 2001)	6–12 (8.8) mm
Midcoronary sinus, cross-sect. area	(Silver and Rowley 1988)	26–58 (38.8) mm^2
	(Silver and Rowley 1988)	29–109 (52.4) mm^{2*}
Atrial ostium, diameter	(Silver and Rowley 1988)	5–14 (8.6) mm
	(Robert 1958)	3–8×5–10 mm
	(Silver and Rowley 1988)	7–16 (9.7) mm*
Atrial ostium, diameter	(Maric et al. 1996)	5–20 mm (8.4 mm)
	(Potkin and Roberts 1987)	4.5–7.3 (6.2) mm
	(Hellerstein and Orbison 1951)	7–19 (9.9) mm
	(Piffer et al. 1990)	5–17 mm
Atrial ostium, cross-sect. area	(Silver and Rowley 1988)	20–154 (61.5) mm^2
	(Silver and Rowley 1988)	38–201 (77.1) mm^{2*}
	(Potkin and Roberts 1987)	16–42 (31) mm^2
Atrial ostium, circumference	(Silver and Rowley 1988)	14–23 (20) mm*
	(Silver and Rowley 1988)	17–53 (35) mm*
Volume1	(Silver and Rowley 1988)	0.7–2.1 (1.26) mm^3
	(Silver and Rowley 1988)	1.0–3.5 (1.76) mm^{3*}

*Results obtained from specimens with increased weight.

A semi-quantitative classification of the length and form was given by Maros et al. (1983):
- A short CS (less than 20 mm) with a compact, bellied form in 11%
- A medium-length CS (20–40 mm) with a narrow, cylindrical form in 74%
- A long CS (60 mm and more) with a tubular, stretched form in 15%

4.4
Diameter, Area of Cross-Section, Circumference, and Volume

These measurements were made by Tandler (1926), Hellerstein and Orbison (1951), Potkin and Roberts (1987), Silver and Rowley (1988), Piffer et al. (1990), and Ortale et al. (2001) on unselected hearts of normal weight (average 351 g) and of increased weight (average 458 g). It was noted (by the various authors) that in patients who had died from chronic congestive heart failure the CS was enlarged, thus the resulting measurements are of a significantly greater magnitude (Fig. 5a–c).

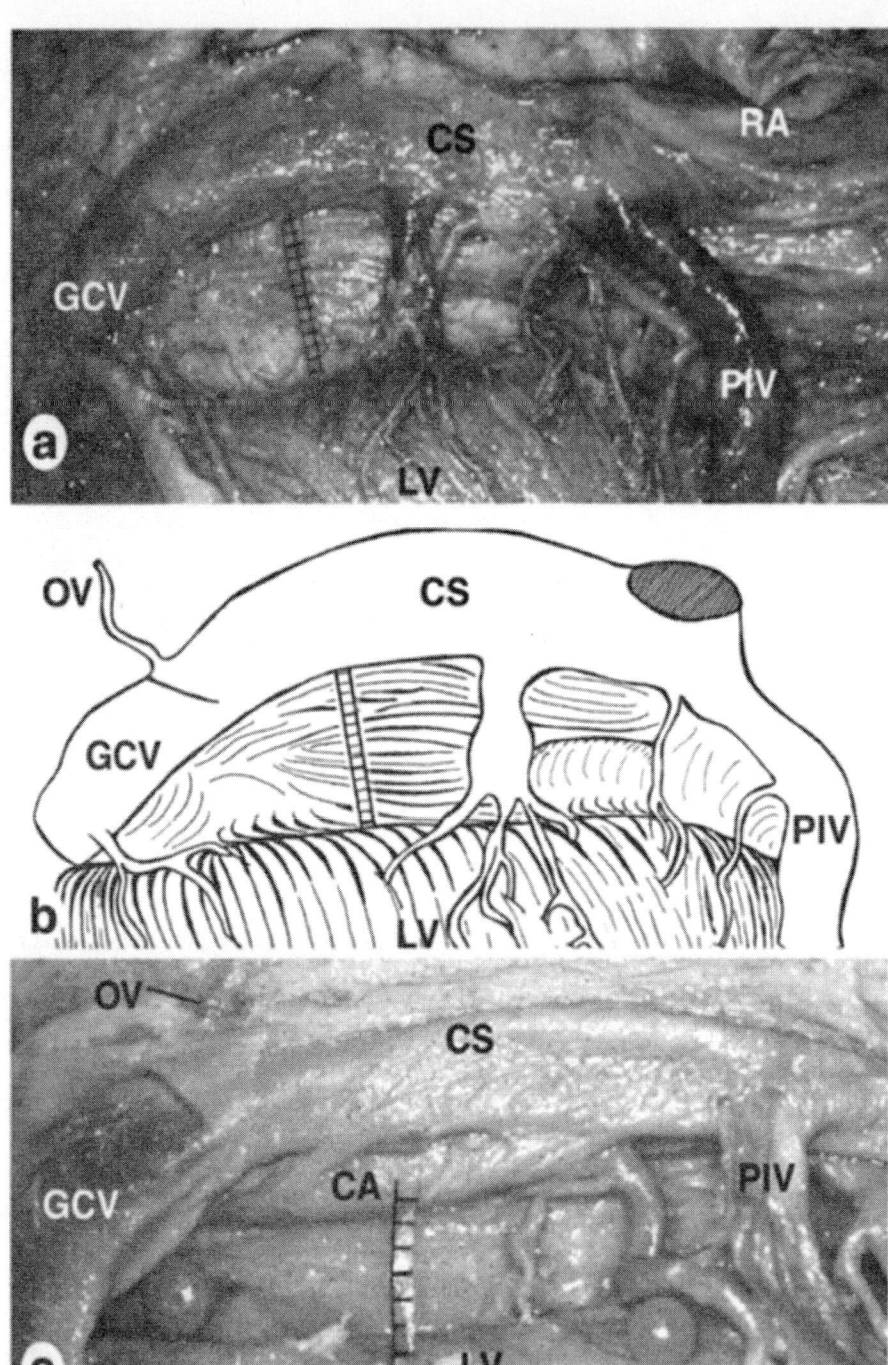

Fig. 5a–c. Grade of elevation of the human CS from the posterior coronary sulcus to the posterior wall of the LA (seen from dorsal). a Severe elevation of the CS to a high position of about 14 mm. b Schematic drawing corresponding to a. c Moderate elevation of the CS to a medium position of about 8 mm. Two small myocardial belts (*white arrows*) originating from the myocardial covering of the CS surround the CA

4.5
Elevation, Curvature, and Ostial Angle

Elevation. Due to a rotation of the heart during lifetime, the CS was more or less displaced from the bottom of the posterior coronary sulcus to the posterior wall of the left atrium. A slight elevation of the CS was found in 12%, a moderate elevation in 50%, and an extreme elevation of up to 15 mm above the bottom of the coronary sulcus with a remarkable arched course in 22% of the cases examined in this study.

The higher the elevation of the CS, the more S-shaped the course of the terminal portion of the GCV appeared to be (von Lüdinghausen and Schott 1990) (Figs. 5a-c) (Table 3).

Curvature. The terminal GCV and its continuation, the CS, describe a gentle curve in the left posterior coronary sulcus or – when the CS is elevated in the manner previously described – on the posterior wall of the LA. The extent of the curvature is determined by three factors: the curvature of the coronary sulcus, the size of the ostial angle of the CS, and the degree of elevation of the CS (von Lüdinghausen and Schott 1990) (Fig. 6a-c) (Table 4).

Ostial Angle. The actual nature of the curvature depends on the size of the ostial angle which, in about half of our cases, was determined by the sharp degree of inner curvature of the terminal CS, and on the absolute length of the CS (von Lüdinghausen and Schott 1990) (Fig. 7).

Table 3. Incidence of the elevation of the CS in the left posterior coronary sulcus

"Normal" position, no elevation	16%
Slight elevation (1–3 mm)	12%
Moderate elevation (4–7 mm)	50%
Extreme elevation (8–15 mm)	22%

Table 4. Curvature of the CS

1/4 of a circle	33%
1/8 of a circle	29%
A gentle curvature	29%
Nearly straight course	9%

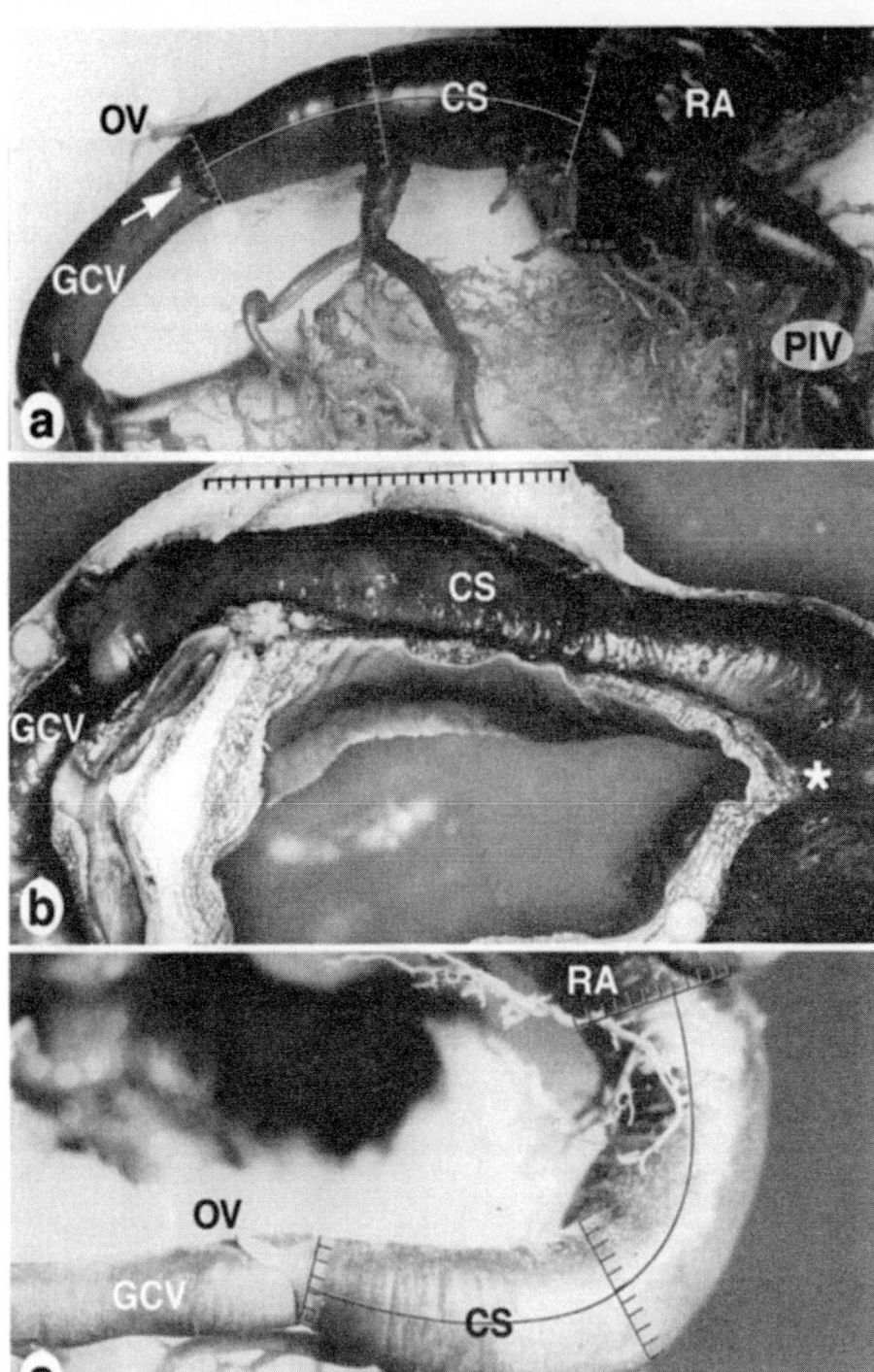

Fig. 6a–c.

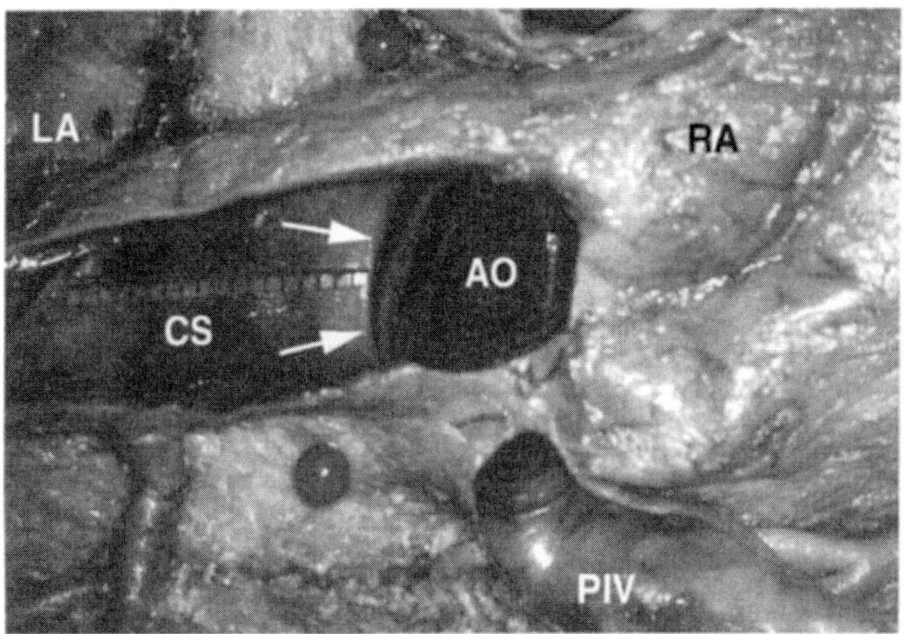

Fig. 7. Longitudinally sectioned CS as seen from dorsal: a pronounced ostial angle (approximately a rectangle) near the ostial opening (*AO*) is marked by *white arrows*

4.6
The Ostial Valve

The oval atrial ostium of the CS is mostly (with a frequency of 81% in our specimens and in 80% according to Parsonnet 1953) provided with a single valve with a concave margin. It closes the ostium more or less completely (Siding 1896; Schippel 1965; Tschabitscher 1986; Silver and Rowley 1988; Piffer et al. 1990) and is highly variable in size and form. The forms range from a complete circular or septal, to an incomplete cribriform, semilunar, crescentic, and threadlike valve. According to Piffer et al. (1990), the length and width of the valve varied in their specimens from 0.2 to 0.9 mm in adults.

In 19% of our cases a real valve was absent (von Lüdinghausen and Schott 1990) (Table 5).

Fig. 6a–c. Curvature and position of the CS, as seen in corrosion casts (a and c) and in a cadaveric specimen (b). a Convex posterior surface of a CS which is about 40 mm long. The diameter at its origin is about 6 mm, at a point halfway along its length it is about 8 mm and the diameter of the ostium about 8 mm. An ostial valve of the GCV is marked by a *white arrow*. b Longitudinally sectioned CS as see from inferior. This case exhibits only a slight curvature. c Superior aspect of a CS with a marked curvature which conforms to a quarter circle. The length of the CS is about 40 mm, its form narrow and cylindrical; the diameter at origin is about 5.5 mm. The diameter at a point about halfway along its length and the diameter of the ostium are both about 10 mm

Table 5. Shape and incidence of the atrial valve of the CS

Complete circular or septal valve (own material)	31%
Hellerstein and Orbison (1951)	30.7%
Silver and Rowley (1988)	20%
Piffer et al. (1990)	9%
Incomplete cribriform valve (own material)	7%
Hellerstein and Orbison (1951)	5.3%
Maric et al. (1996)	12.5%
Incomplete semilunar valve (own material)	7%
Hellerstein and Orbison (1951)	6%
Piffer et al. (1990)	30%
Incomplete crescentic valve (own material)	34%
Hellerstein and Orbison (1951)	38%
Incomplete thread-like valve (own material)	2%
Hellerstein and Orbison (1951)	5.3%
Valveless orifice	
Mochizuki (1933)	3%
Wright et al. (1948)	20%
Hellerstein and Orbison (1951)	14.7%
Sarrazin (1965)	29%
Schippel (1965)	11%
Silver and Rowley (1988)	16%
Maric et al. (1996)	10%
Piffer et al. (1990)	30%
(Own material)	19%
Complete congenital atresia (own material)	1%
Giebel et al. (2000)	0.5%

The valve of the CS, the ostial valve of the IVC, and the crista terminalis are generally regarded as derivatives or remnants of the right valve of the sinus venosus (Yater 1929; Wright et al. 1948) (Figs. 8a–c, 9a–d).

Schippel (1965) and Piffer et al. (1990) found the diameter of an oval CS orifice to vary from 2 to 7 mm in the smaller range, and from 12 to 17 mm in the larger range, irrespective of the presence or absence of an ostial valve. Annular myocardial tissue was found to encircle the atrial orifice of the CS, and some valves were thick and fleshy (Schippel 1965). The smallest thickness of the valve was 25 nm, the greatest 1.4 mm. Histological examination revealed that the valvular stroma of cases examined by both Schippel (1965) and Piffer (1990) contained myocardial fibers deriving from the myocardial coat; such fibers were even found in the threads of a cribriform valve. The purpose of the sphincter-like annular musculature surrounding the orifice and the muscle fibers in the valvular stroma is to support the ostial valve in closing the ostium and preventing a reflow during atrial presystole (according to Piffer et al. 1990).

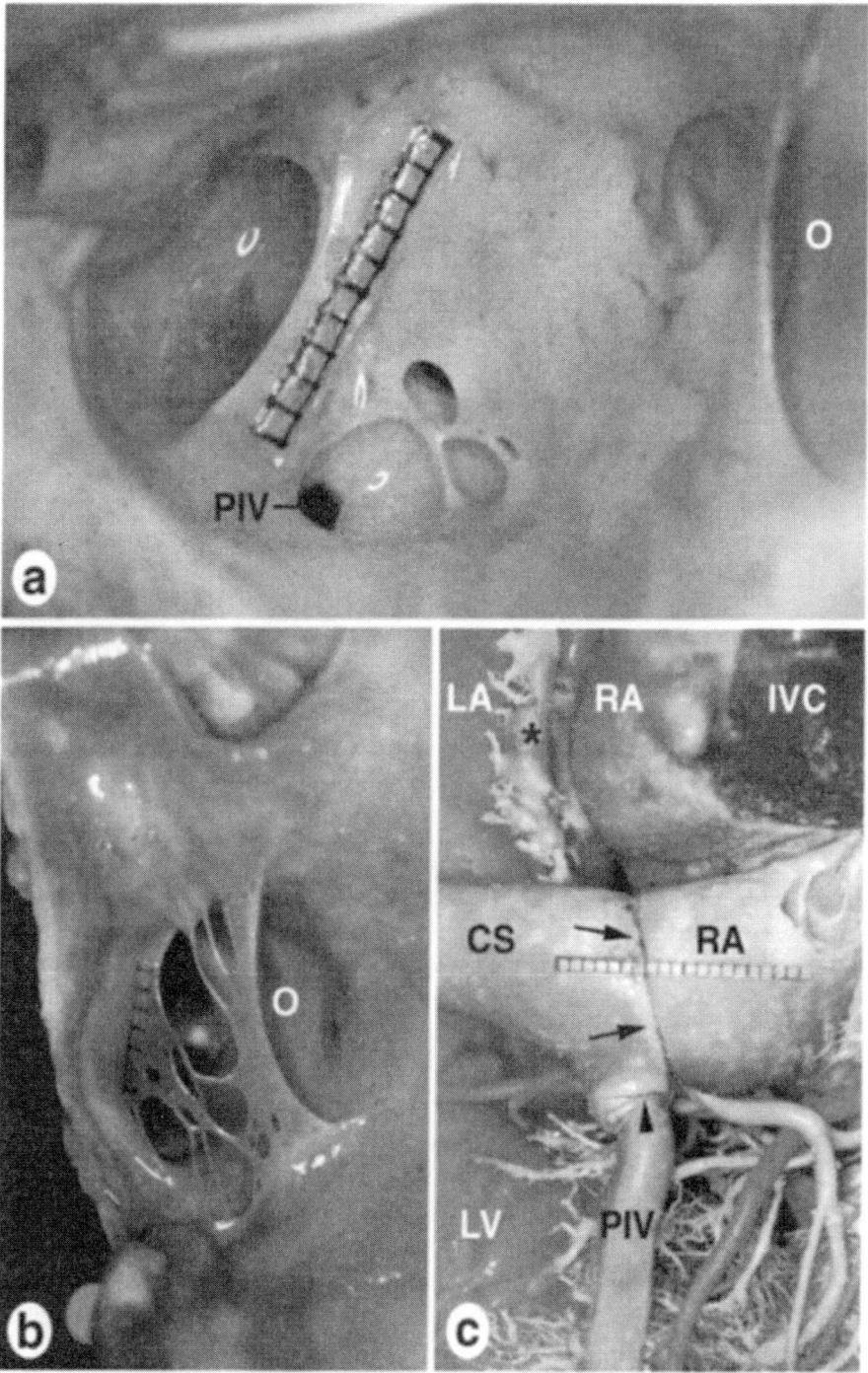

Fig. 8a–c. Various forms of the ostial valve of the CS as seen in cadaveric specimens (a and b) and in a corrosion cast (c). a An incomplete valve with a perforated leaflet. The atrial ostium of the CS is marked (O); the opening of the PIV is also indicated. b A cribriform valve. c Posterior view of the crux cordis region showing an impression left by the ostial valves of the CS and the PIV (marked by *black arrows*). Also visible is an intramural venous sinus (marked by an *asterisk*) in the interatrial septum. The former presumably collects atrial veins and then opens into the RA

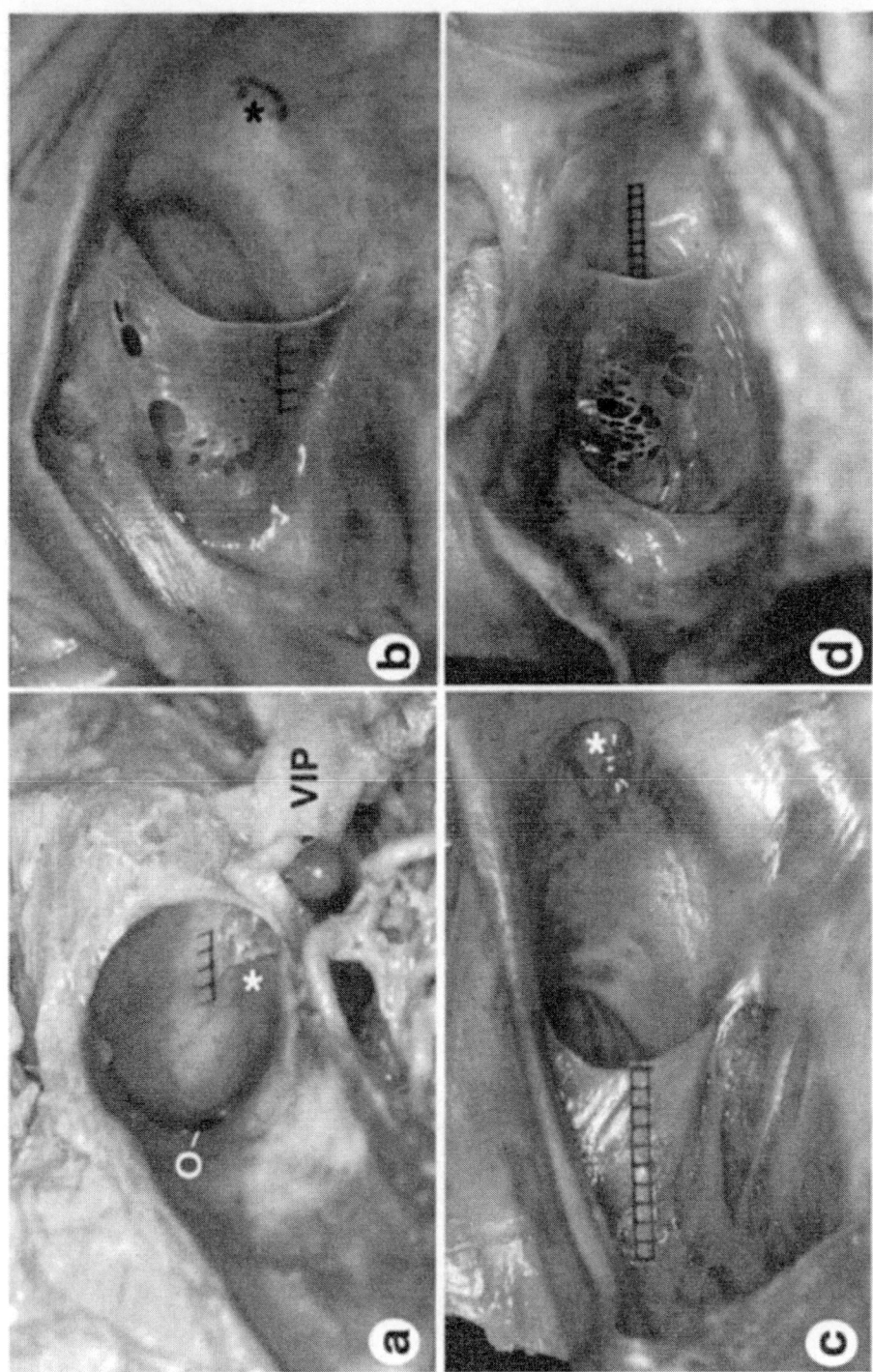

Fig. 9a–d.

4.7
Enlargement of the CS, Aneurysm of the CS

In rare cases, dilation and aneurysm-like magnification of the CS may occur, mimicking an intrapericardial compact tumor. Wenger and Zandanell (1969) described such an aneurysm 5×5×2 cm in size and almost full of tough, old clots.

4.8
Enlargement of the CS Associated
with Persistent Left Superior Vena Cava

A fairly common variation is that the left SVC remains persistent and terminates in the left aspect of the CS. Given this circumstance, the significance of the CS increases because it drains not only cardiac veins but also the blood from the left SVC. Accordingly, it is greatly enlarged (Vlodaver et al. 1976).

4.9
Enlargement of the CS Associated with Ostial Occlusion

Symptomless atresia of the atrial ostium of the CS in an adult heart specimen, combined with a persistent left SVC (Cuvieri's duct) but no other cardiac anomalies or malformations, is a rare finding (Siding 1896; Hutton 1915; Peele 1932; Reed 1938/1939; Mantini et al. 1966; Frank and Maloney 1968; Gerlis et al. 1984; von Lüdinghausen and Lechleuthner 1988; Giebel et al. 2000). Such an atrial occlusion of the CS by a thick, smooth membrane is undoubtedly congenital in origin and may thus be designated an atresia (Edwards 1960).

According to Bankl (1977), four types of occlusion have been observed: (1) with the left SVC draining retrograde to the left brachiocephalic vein, (2) with a large connection to the left atrium, (3) with multiple connections via Thebesian vessels to the atria, and (4) with a leviatrio-cardinal vein connecting the CS and LA.

- The instance of ostial occlusion (atresia) of the CS, described by von Lüdinghausen and Lechleuthner (1988), belongs – in accordance with Bankl (1977) - partly to type 1 and partly to type 3 (Fig. 10a,b).

Therefore we can assume the possibility of the existence of variations exhibiting the characteristics of a combination of the groups.

Fig. 9a–d. Various forms of the ostial valve of the CS as seen in cadaveric specimens. **a** A complete membranous ostial valve, seen through the opened CS. The atrial ostium is marked (O). The ostium of the posterior interventricular vein (indicated by a *white asterisk*) is integrated into the leaflet of the ostial valve of the CS. **b** An incomplete crescentic, perforated ostial valve of the CS. The ostium of an intramural sinus which drains the myocardium of the inferior interatrial septum is indicated by an *asterisk*. **c** An incomplete crescentic, unperforated ostial valve of the CS. The opening of the sinus of the interatrial septum is indicated by an *asterisk*. **d** An incomplete, cribriform ostial valve of the CS. The atrial opening is marked by a *millimeter scale*

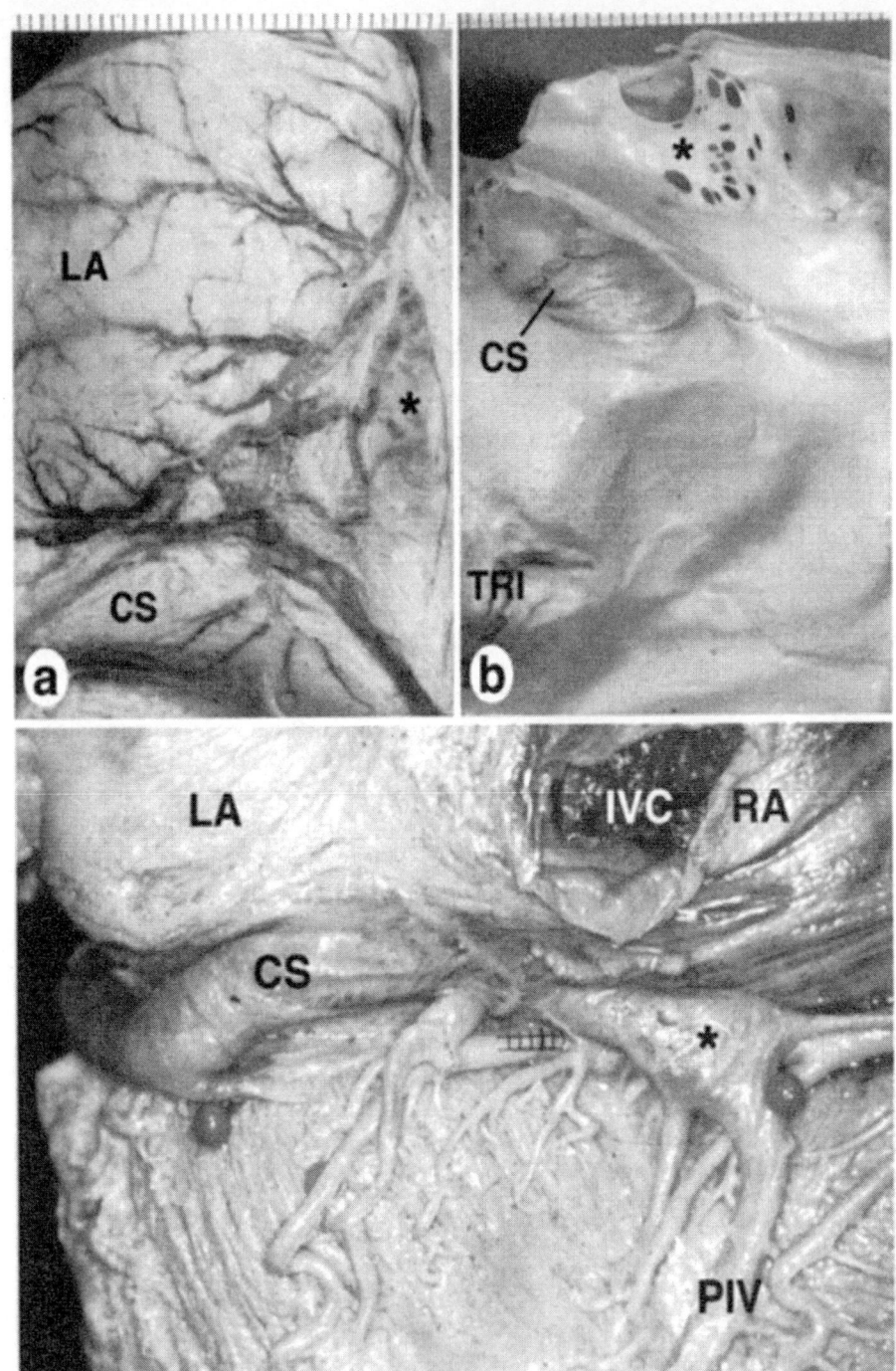

Fig. 10a–c.

4.10
Duplication of the CS (Sinus Coronarius 'Duplex')

In very rare cases the terminal oblique part of the PIV in the crux cordis area just beneath the opening of the IVC appeared widened and enlarged, with a diameter which was almost as large as that of the CS. It was covered by myocardial fibers in the same way as the CS.

Because of its similarity to a (short) CS, it was designated a "duplication" of the CS, accessory CS, or sinus coronarius "duplex" (von Lüdinghausen et al. 1994) (Fig. 10c).

4.11
Absence of the CS

Cases in which the CS is completely absent and the cardiac veins drain separately into the left and right atria were classified by Mantini et al. (1966) as exhibiting (1) a septal defect of the atrium localized in the position normally occupied by the CS, and (2) a septal defect of the atrium involving the entire lower portion of the septum with a persistent common atrioventricular canal or with asplenia and congenital cardiac disease.

Bankl (1977) and Foale et al. (1979) also revealed that the absence of a CS is never an isolated anomaly; it is always associated with a persistent left SVC. However, Bergman et al. (1988) dissected a heart specimen in which a CS was absent and where the GCV was found to pass upward, cross the coronary sulcus beneath the left coronary artery, course through the transverse epicardial sinus, and empty into the (right) SVC. The other veins of the diaphragmatic and anterior surface of the heart, including the marginal vein and SCV, drained into the right atrium through an ostium protected by a smooth valve.

Fig. 10a–c. Peculiarities of the CS as seen in human heart specimens. a Posterior wall of the LA showing numerous atrial veins which empty into an intramural venous sinus of the posterior part of the interatrial septum (marked by an *asterisk*). The sinus opens into the RA. The atrial veins function as anastomoses between the CS and the RA in a case of ostial occlusion or ostial atresia of the CS. However, in this case the main venous drainage of the myocardium is effected by a persisting left superior vena cava. The intramural venous sinus of the interatrial septum above the occlusion is indicated by a *black asterisk*. b Interior aspect of the RA (the same specimen as in a) exhibiting the membranous occlusion of the CS. Parts of the tricuspid valve can be seen below the occlusion. c A so-called sinus coronarius duplex (duplicate coronary sinus) (marked by an *asterisk*) is situated inferior to the ostium of the IVC. This "right" CS is formed from a widened oblique part of the terminal PIV and empties directly into the RA

5
The Myocardial Cover of the Coronary Sinus and Related Veins

5.1
The Myocardial Cover of the CS

In commonly used textbooks and atlases (Töndury 1970; Platzer 1982; Fleischhauer 1985; Leonhardt 1987; Putz and Pabst 2000) the myocardial coat of the CS is either not depicted or it is inaccurately documented.

Our meticulous dissection of all the human heart specimens revealed that the CS was wrapped in a thin layer of myocardial fibers constituting a muscular wall or myocardial coat which appeared to be less than 1 mm thick. The fibers of this coat were firmly attached to, and intermingled with, the myocardial fibers from the posteroinferior wall of the left atrium.

Superficially the fibers were arranged in spirals or followed - along the total length of the CS - a longitudinal, an oblique, or an axially orientated course. During dissection, "left atrial" myocardial muscle fibers frequently required division. Therefore, the CS is located intramurally and is an integrated part of the left atrial myocardium, a point which should be stressed. This myocardial right-left duality will not be deemed singular if the origin of the CS from the left horn of the sinus venosus is recalled (McAlpine 1975; Maros et al. 1983; Waller and Schlant 1994).

In all cases studied, the proximal and distal edges of this coat of the CS are irregular and not sharply defined; it appeared to be impossible to measure the exact length of the CS from outside (von Lüdinghausen et al. 1992) (Figs. 3a–c, 5a–c, 11a–d).

5.1.1
Peculiarity

In one case the circumflex branch of the left coronary artery coursed in very close relationship to the GCV and CS; its terminal part was also wrapped in the myocardial coat of the CS (von Lüdinghausen et al. 1992).

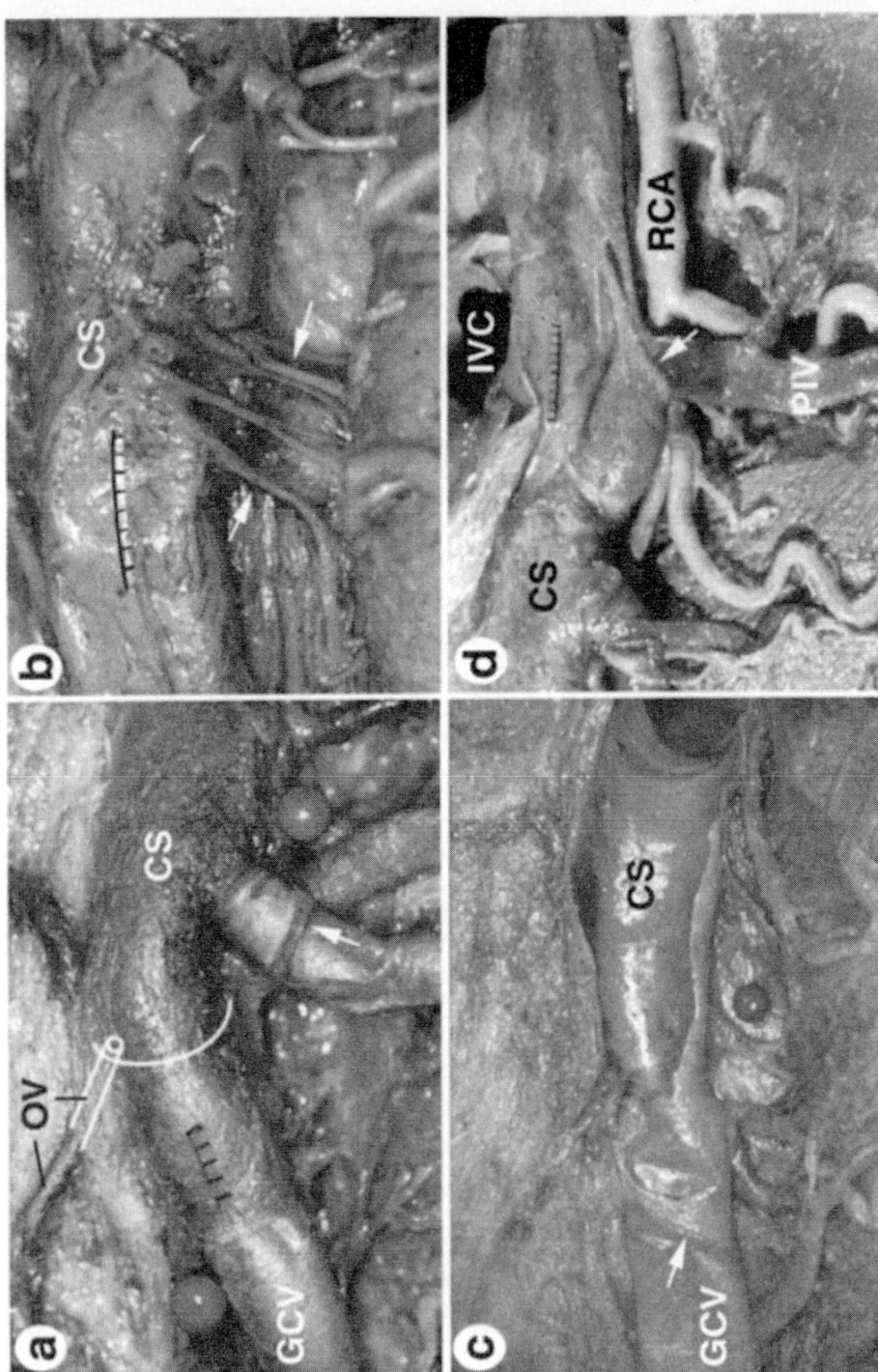

Fig. 11a–d.

5.2
The Left (Distal) Boundary of the Myocardial Coat of the CS
and the Myocardial Cuff of the Terminal GCV

5.2.1
The Myocardial Coat of the CS

The reason for the lack of sharp definition of the distal edge/boundary of the myocardial coat of the CS was that, in almost all cases examined, the myocardial coat was longer than the CS itself. In all cases the coat spread over the beginning of the CS, which is marked by the opening of the OV, and extended to the left to cover the terminal part of the GCV (Figs. 11a–c, 12a–c).

5.2.2
The Myocardial Cuff of the Terminal GCV

In doing so, the myocardial coat of the CS formed a peripheral myocardial cuff surrounding the distal GCV, and averaged 3.6 mm (1–11 mm) in length. The obliquely coursing fiber bundles of the cuff changed direction and surrounded the vein in a belt- or sphincter-like fashion. In 15% of these heart specimens the cuffs were thickened, which caused the narrowing of the terminal portion of the GCV to a variable degree.

The left boundary or edge of the myocardial coat of the CS is formed by fibers in such a way as to exhibit a straight, oblique, or crescent-shaped margin, or the fibers are arranged diffusely (von Lüdinghausen et al. 1992). This latter, diffuse dispersion is demonstrated in an excellent illustration by Pernkopf (1937).

There were four different orientations of the left myocardial fibers. In 58% of (our) cases, obliquely coursing fibers of the coat ran parallel to the course of the OV. In 19% the marginal fibers crossed the great vein at right angles, and in 9% a crescent-like pattern was seen. In 14% the edge of the myocardial coat was ill-defined with a splitting-up of the fibers (von Lüdinghausen et al. 1992) (Figs. 11a–c, 12a,b).

Fig. 11a–d. Peculiarities of the myocardial coverage of the CS and related veins as seen on the posterior wall of the LV in cadaveric specimens: **a** The myocardial coat of the CS extends to the terminal part of the GCV (indicated by a *scale*). The presumed position of the ostial valve of the GCV is indicated by a *white curved line*. The opening of the OV into the CS is also indicated and marks the exact beginning of the CS. A small myocardial belt (indicated by a *white arrow*) encircles the terminal PVLV. **b** A CS in a moderately elevated position on the dorsal wall of the left atrium. A few isolated myocardial fiber cords arise from the inferior wall of the CS and dip downwards to the posterior coronary sulcus and adjacent ventricular myocardium. **c** An isolated myocardial belt (indicated by a *white arrow*) encircles the terminal portion of the GCV (opened CS). **d** The crux cordis region below the atrial ostium of the IVC and adjacent to the myocardial coverage of the distal part of the CS: the terminal oblique part of the PIV is also encircled by myocardial stripes (*arrow*) and fixed by myocardial cords to the posterior wall of the RA. The PIV crosses, as usual, over the RCA

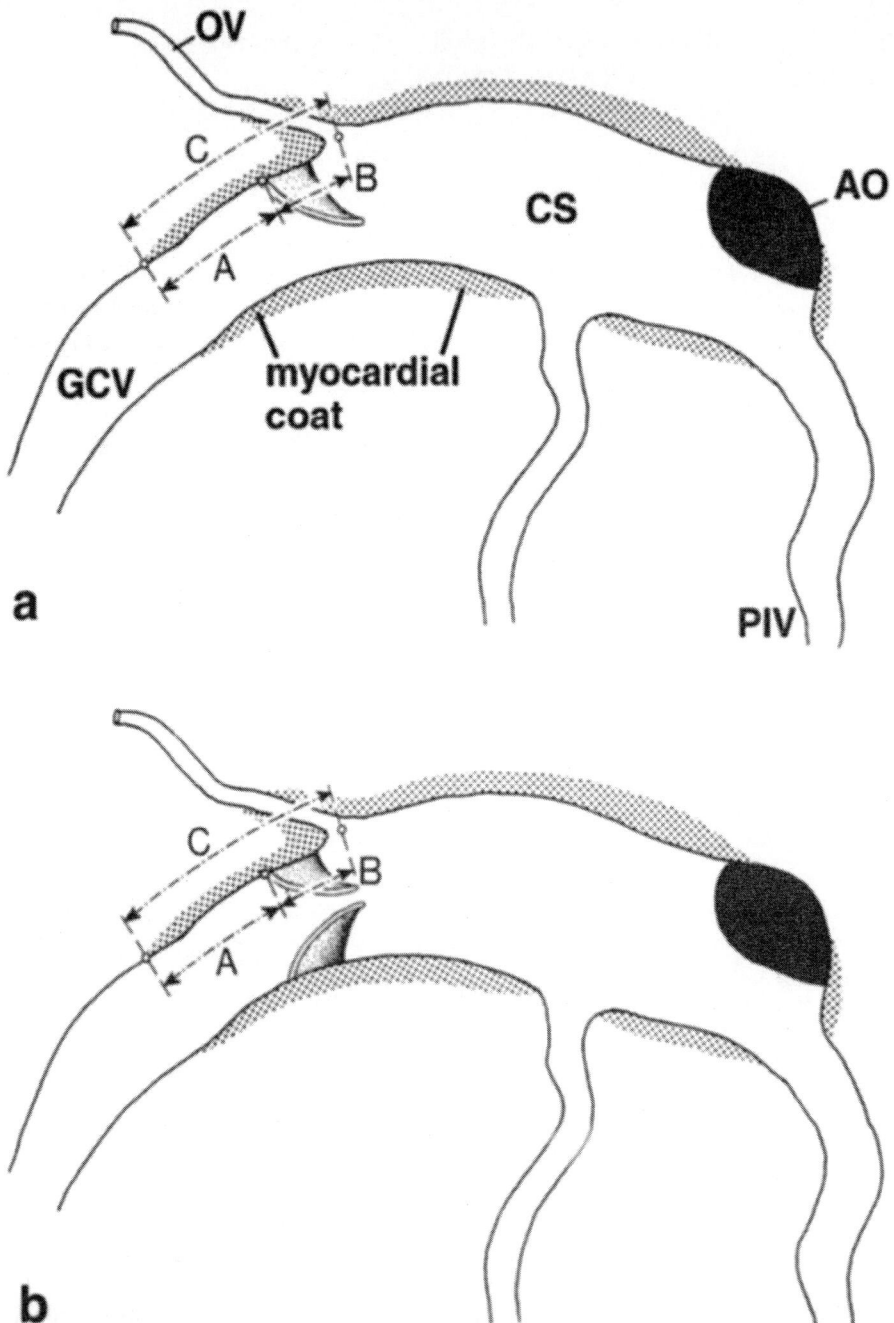

Fig. 12a, b. Diagram of the opened CS, showing a unicuspid (a) and a bicuspid (b) valve of the GCV, and landmarks at the transient zone of GCV and CS. The distance *A* denotes the distance between the left free edge of the myocardial cuff and the attachment of the valve of the GCV. The distance *B* denotes the distance between the valve of the GCV and the opening of the OV. The distance *C* indicates the distance between the free edge of the myocardial cuff and the opening of the OV. All distances are highly variable and are not appropriate to determine the length of the CS. There are arguments for the thesis that only the opening of the OV marks the true beginning of the CS

5.3
The Right (Proximal) Boundary of the Myocardial Coat of the CS

The myocardial fiber bundles of the myocardial coat of the terminal CS ran parallel to the coronary sulcus and continued into the posteroinferior wall of the right atrium. In 3% of the hearts studied, some fiber bundles extended to the adjacent terminal (oblique) part of the PIV and to the SCV. The terminal part of the latter was often widened just before entry into the CS.

In 5% of the cases studied, the myocardial coat of the terminal (oblique) portion of the PIV fastened the vein to the dorsal right atrial wall (von Lüdinghausen et al. 1992) (Figs. 12d, 13).

5.4
Isolated Myocardial Belts in the Terminal Portions of Other Cardiac Veins

In addition to the frequent finding of a myocardial cuff around a number of cardiac veins as described above, there were also one or two isolated myocardial belts surrounding the GCV and/or the posterior vein of the left ventricle. The belts were found in 9% of the cases we examined, averaged 4 mm in breadth, and exhibited no connection to the myocardial coat or cuffs of the CS previously described. In 2% of these cases, such isolated belts were seen to surround both the GCV and PVLV. In 5% only the terminal portion of the GCV was surrounded by one or two isolated myocardial belts; in 1% there was a partly separated belt. In the remaining 2% of these cases, a few small myocardial fibers formed an isolated myocardial belt surrounding only the PVLV (von Lüdinghausen and Schott 1990; von Lüdinghausen et al. 1992) (Table 6) (Figs. 11c, 13).

Table 6. Occurrence of myocardial coats, cuffs, and belts in connection with the cover of the CS (own material)

Terminal great cardiac vein with a cuff of 1–3 mm width	80%
Great cardiac vein with a cuff of 4–8 mm width	18%
Great cardiac vein with a cuff of 8–11 mm width	2%
Occurrence of accessory isolated myocardial belts of the Great cardiac vein	5%
Posterior vein of the left ventricle alone	2%
Great cardiac vein and posterior vein of the left ventricle	2%

5.5
"Free" Myocardial Cords
in the Left Posterior Coronary Sulcus

In 8% of our cases, one or several small myocardial cords originated from the myocardial tissue covering the inferior wall of the CS and passed freely through the adipose tissue of the posterior coronary groove. After traveling 9–12 mm, they dipped downwards into the superficial myocardial layer of the posteroinferior left atrial wall, thereafter running to the outer circumference of the fibrous mitral ring or – most surprisingly – to the adjacent ventricular myocardium. In 6% of cases, myocardial fiber cords surrounded the terminal circumflex branch of the left coronary artery and fixed it to the dorsal wall of the left atrial myocardium (von Lüdinghausen and Schott 1990; von Lüdinghausen et al. 1992).

Patients with direct atrioventricular myocardial connections consisting of bundles of myocardial muscle fibers in the coronary sulcus (anomalous atrioventricular muscle bundle or Kent bundle) may exhibit ventricular pre-excitation, for instance Wolff–Parkinson–White (WPW) syndrome (Rosen et al. 1980; Rigby and Graboys 1981; Sealy and Mikat 1983; Robinson et al. 1988) (Figs. 11b, 13).

5.6
The Proximal Origin of the CS and Its Landmarks

Three anatomical landmarks are currently recognized for the origin of the CS: the left margin of the myocardial covering of the CS, the valve of the GCV, and the junction of the OV and the CS. These landmarks are imprecise, being distributed over an area of up to 12 mm.

In one-third of the cases, the three landmarks were found close together within an area 2–4 mm in length, in another third they were distributed over an area 5–8 mm in length, and in the remaining cases the area of distribution was 9–12 mm in length. These so-called landmarks were found in the posterior coronary sulcus, with the peripheral edge of the myocardial cover located to the left of them, the valve of the GCV in the middle, and the opening of the OV to the right (von Lüdinghausen et al. 1992).

Because the myocardial covering of the CS continued in a leftward direction over towards the adjacent great vein for an average distance of 6 mm, its sometimes ill-defined left margin prevented its use as a point of origin. The broad attachment of cusps or leaflets over an area of 1–6 mm likewise rendered the valve of the GCV unsuitable as a point from which measurements concerning the anatomical beginning of the CS can be made. Furthermore, the valve of the GCV was found only in 87% of our specimens, and the number of cusps varied from one (in 62% of cases) to two (in 25%) and even three (less than 1%). The dot-like opening of the OV (found in 95% of the cases) was such a constant feature that it represented the point from which measurements could carefully be carried out (Figs. 12a,b, 13).

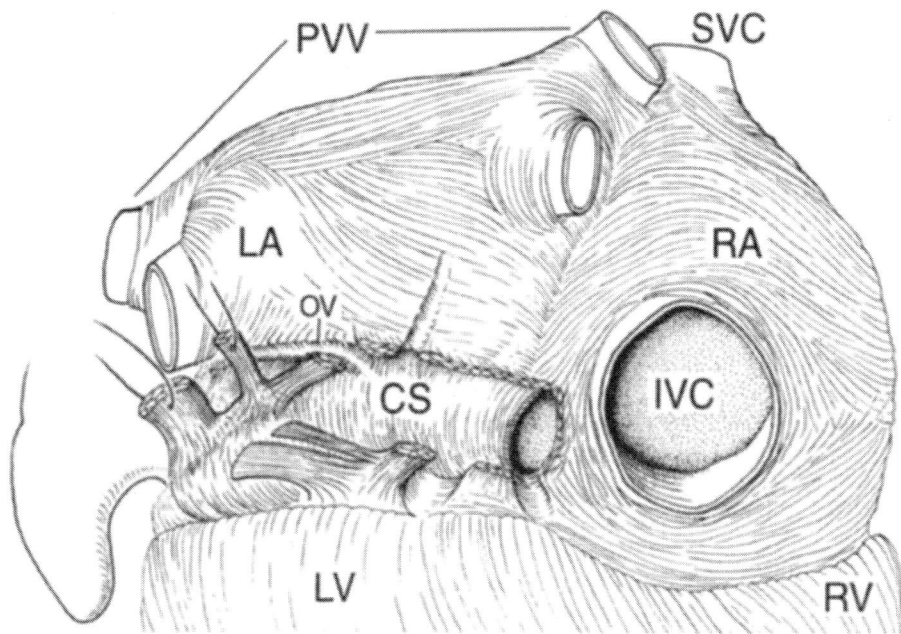

Fig. 13. Schematic drawing of the posterior wall of both atria. The cut edges of the myocardial coat and belts of the CS and related veins are visible after removal of the vascular tube of the CS. The myocardial fiber bundles of the coat and belts derive from the walls of the left atrium and from the posterior coronary sulcus

5.6.1
The OV Is the Only Exact Peripheral Landmark for the Origin of the CS

In recent textbooks and atlases, reference has been made to one, two, or three landmarks for the origin of the CS: (1) the peripheral edge of the myocardial coat on the surface of the CS, (2) the opening of the OV, and (3) the terminal valve of the GCV (Tandler 1913; McAlpine 1975; Tschabitscher 1984, Putz and Pabst 2000). These structures were held to be safe and reliable external and internal landmarks for the exact determination of the beginning of the CS.

However, structures in the left posterior sulcus were found by von Lüdinghausen et al. (1992) to be unreliable and useless where definition of the conjunction of the GCV and the CS is concerned, because they extended over an area 2–6 mm in length, in the following sequence from left to right: the myocardial cuff of the terminal part of the GCV (a continuation of the myocardial coat of the CS), the valve of the GCV with an attachment 1–6 mm in width, and the dot-like opening of the OV.

The opening of the OV and the ostial valve of the GCV were found to be separated by an average distance of 2.5 mm; this has also been noticed in studies of corrosion casts (Tschabitscher 1986). The average distance between the broad attachment of the valve of the GCV and the peripheral left edge of the myocardial coat was about 6 mm. This peripheral left edge was formed in such a way as to exhibit straight, oblique, or crescent-shaped margins, or a diffuse arrangement of the fibers.

In conclusion, and also in terms of embryological development, the opening of the OV is the only logical and safe landmark.

5.6.2
Clinical Significance of Accessory Myocardial Cuffs, Belts, and Cords

The myocardial coat of the CS, the myocardial cuffs of the terminal parts of the adjoining ventricular veins, and the isolated myocardial belts and cords in the depths of the posterior left coronary sulcus can constitute accessory atrioventricular connections and in this respect epicardial posteroseptal and left posterior atrioventricular accessory pathways of the conduction system, designated as Kent's bundles (Becker et al. 1978; Schneider and Kappenberger 1980; Cox and Ferguson 1989; von Lüdinghausen et al. 1992; Sun et al. 2002).

Clinically, this phenomenon might be related to some forms of WPW syndrome (Rigby and Graboys 1981). The oblique orientation of the myocardial fibers connecting the CS coat with the left atrium and sometimes with the left ventricle would explain the usually oblique course of these accessory pathways.

The objective of surgery for the WPW syndrome is to divide the accessory atrioventricular connection (accessory pathway) responsible for the syndrome (Cox and Ferguson 1989).

6 The Anatomy of the Veins Draining the Myocardium of Both Ventricles

6.1
The Ventricular Cardiac Veins in General

An extensive intercommunicating network of subepicardially distributed veins provides venous drainage for the coronary circulation (Parsonnet 1953; Waller and Schlant 1994). The ventricular cardiac veins are situated in the epicardium and are therefore easily dissectible throughout most of their course (Figs. 13, 27).

6.1.1
The Apical Venous Network

Ventricular cardiac veins develop from a wide and dense apical venous network, from which four axially orientated venous stems originate. Two of these stems (AIV and PIV) course in the anterior and posterior IV grooves; a further two stems (right and left marginal veins) run along the right and left margins in the direction of the coronary sulcus. Here they empty into the CS or into the dominant vein of the right coronary sulcus. In the case of the anterior left part of the coronary sulcus the dominant vessel is the GCV, in that of the posterior part of the coronary sulcus it is the CS itself, and in that of the right part of the coronary sulcus it is the SCV (Fig. 27).

6.1.2
Venous Valves

Ventricular veins exhibit mostly insufficient uni-, bi-, or tricuspid valves in two locations: (1) at their openings into greater stems and (2) at their openings into the dominant veins of the coronary sulcus (Lechleuthner 1987).

The openings of the cardiac veins entering the CS are marked by uni- or bicuspid valves which, in most of our specimens, appeared to be insufficient. In about one half of our cases these valves were in the ostium itself, in the other half the valves were situated next to the ostia, i.e., at a distance of 1–15 mm near, or distal to, the ostia. This means that, in the latter instance, the terminal venous portion is anatomically and functionally included in the space of the CS (von Lüdinghausen 1987).

6.1.3
Left and Right Ventricular Veins

In the LV and RV, large cardiac veins drain only the external two thirds or three quarters of the myocardium; the internal third or quarter is drained by tributaries of the SCVS (see Chaps. 2.1 "The Greater Cardiac Venous System" and 2.2 "The Smaller Cardiac Venous System").

6.1.4
Left and Right Atrial Veins

In the LA, the myocardium is predominantly drained by delicate cardiac veins which nevertheless belong to the GCVS. In the RA, the walls of the sinus venosus are drained by tributaries of the GCVS; the myocardium of the auricle, however, is mainly drained by tributaries of the SCVS.

6.2
Frequency and Distribution Pattern of the Tributaries of the CS

The primary tributaries of the CS are as follows: the GCV, the left marginal vein, the PVLV, and the PIV. In 30% of the cases studied, the right marginal vein and its terminal part in the right coronary sulcus, the SCV, are tributaries of the CS (Lechleuthner and von Lüdinghausen 1986) (Fig. 14).

For clinical purposes, for instance where selective reperfusion of a single cardiac vein is necessary, it is important to know the frequency of occurrence with which the cardiac veins reach the CS:

- In 11% of the hearts studied, the CS was found to collect all the cardiac veins, i.e., the AIV and the GCV, the LMV, the PVLV, the PIV, the SCV, the RMV, and the ACVs (with the exception of the conal vein and the vein of Zuckerkandl) from the walls of both the left and right ventricles, in equal measure.
- In 25% of the cases the ACVs did not drain into the CS, but connected directly with the RA; the SCV and the RMV into the CS. This situation has been described in most textbooks as constituting the most frequent and typical venous behavior (Lechleuthner and von Lüdinghausen 1986; Williams et al. 1995; Feneis and Dauber 1998).
- In 61% of the cases studied the ACVs, including the RMV from which the SCV originated at the right margin, did not reach the CS, but directly entered the RA.
- In 2% of the cases only the GCV and the PVLV joined the CS; here, all the other veins belonged to the system of the ACVs and opened directly into the RA.
- In 1% of the cases there was an aberrant course of the AIV.

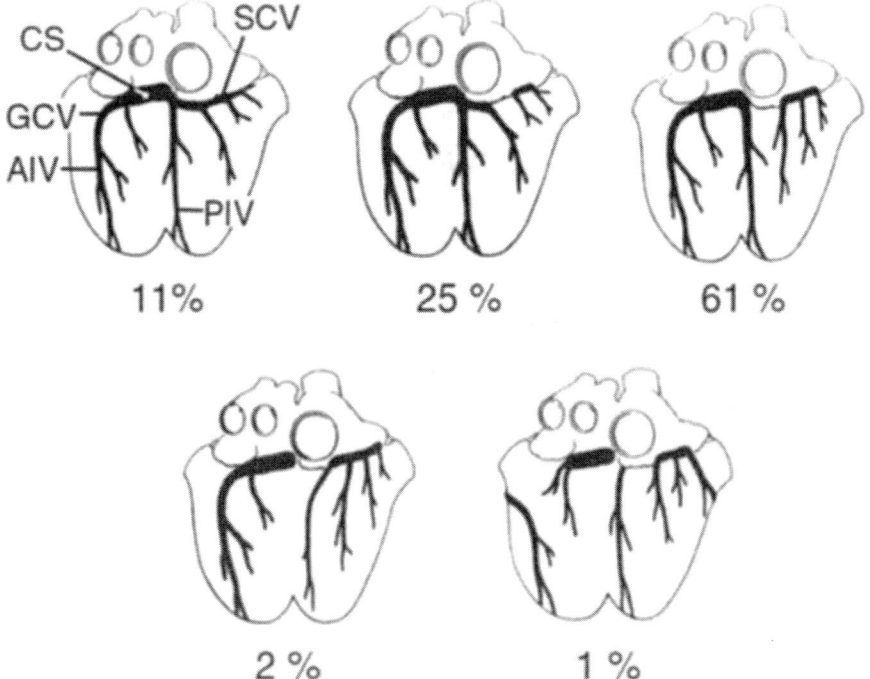

Fig. 14. Schematic two-dimensional drawings of a heart showing the percentages of the many variations in the distribution pattern of the major cardiac veins and the mode of their termination into the CS or directly into the RA

6.3
The Great Cardiac Vein
and the Anterior Interventricular Vein

The GCV existed in all specimens examined by Parsonnet (1953), Pejkovic and Bogdanovic (1992), and Maric et al. (1996), and in 99% of our cases. In general, the tributaries of the GCV are the veins that drain the anterior walls of both ventricles, the apical region, and parts of the IV septum and LA.

The GCV may be divided into two main parts: (1) the AIV and (2) the GCV.
1. The AIV begins as a rather small branch deriving from the dense subepicardial venous network at the apex of the heart; it courses upwards in the anterior IV groove until it reaches the left coronary sulcus and, thereafter, the area of division of the stem of the left coronary artery. It subsequently turns off to the left (Figs. 15, 16a,b).
2. The GCV is designated the longest venous vessel of the heart (Pejkovics and Bogdanovic 1992), constituting a continuation of the AIV. As the GCV proper (a large and thick vessel) it enters the left coronary sulcus, coursing along with the left circumflex artery to the LCM, where it empties into the CS.

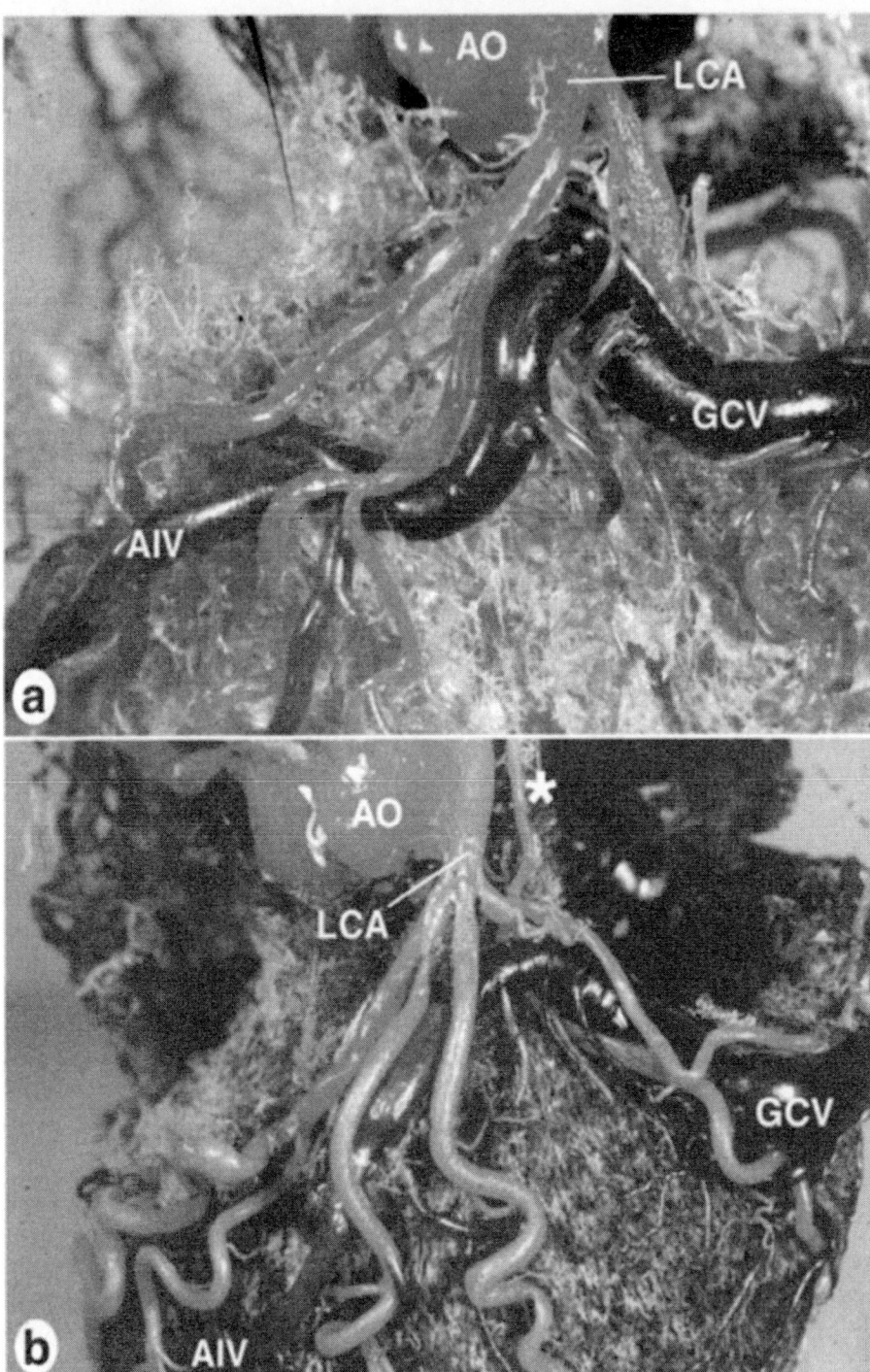

Fig. 15a,b. Relationships between the GCV and the branches of the LCA as seen in corrosion casts. a The GCV passes beneath the AIA and crosses over the CA. b The GCV passes beneath all the branches of the LCA

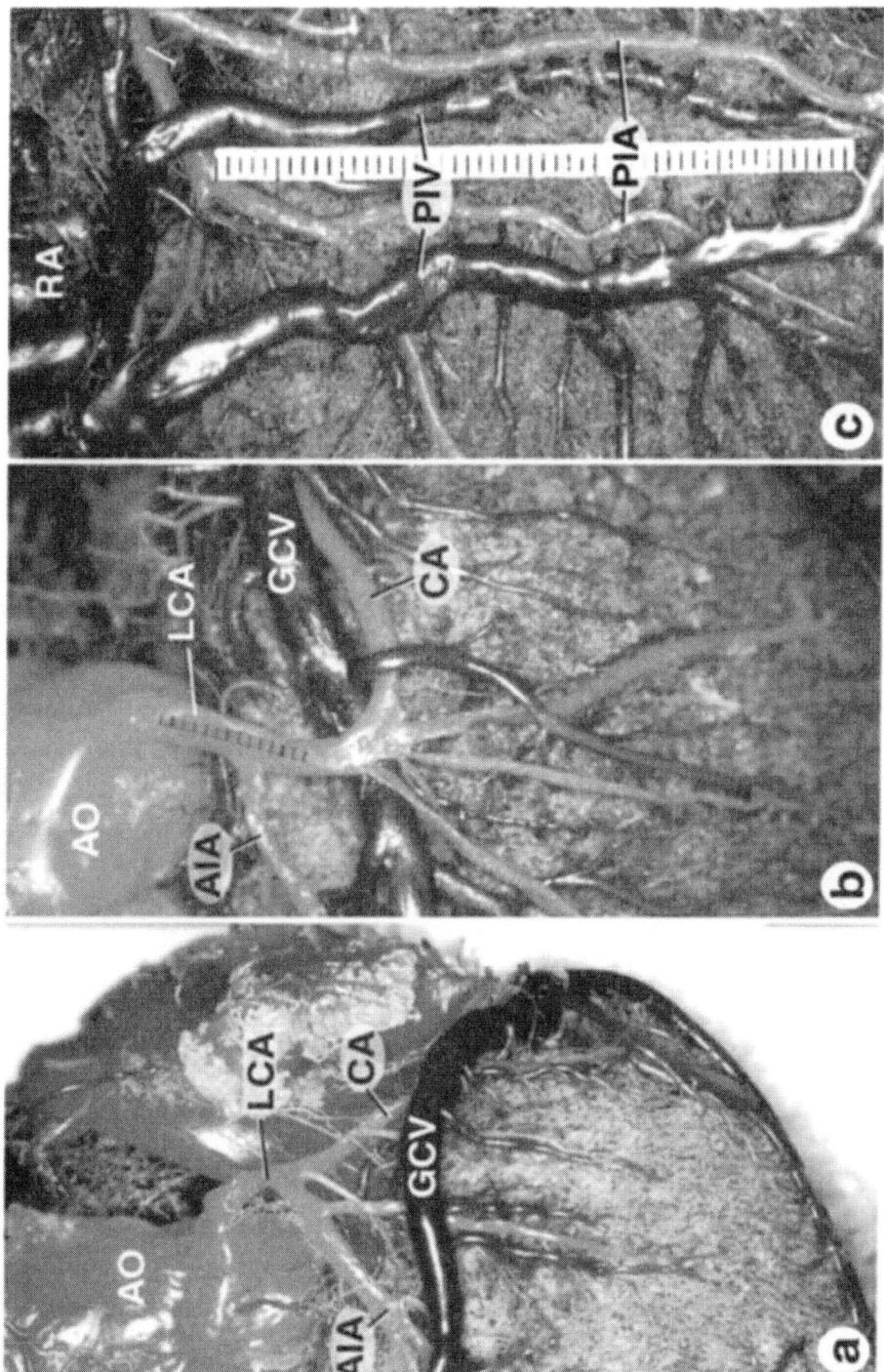

Fig. 16a–c. Relationships between the GCV and the branches of the LCA (a and b) and between the PIV and the PIA as seen in corrosion casts. a The GCV passes over all branches of the LCA. b The GCV passes beneath the CA. c The double PIV passes over the duplicate PIA

Examination of the junction area of the anterior IV sulcus and the left coronary sulcus revealed that the GCV crossed over or under the left circumflex artery or the main stem of the left coronary artery; this behavior will be described later (see Sect. 6.18 "The Relationships Between Cardiac Veins and Coronary Arteries").

Peculiarities

In a few of the cases we examined (8%) extensive compression of the AIV or the GCV seemed to have been caused by its crossing sclerosed or calcified segments of the main stem or branches of the left coronary artery.

In one exception (see Sect. 8.3.12 "Ectopic Origin and Aberrant Course of the AIV"), the AIV did not continue into the GCV when it left the anterior IV sulcus, but turned to the right and crossed the conus arteriosus to become a unique, large ACV (von Lüdinghausen 1989).

In a few cases there was duplication of the AIV; each of these veins accompanied the anterior interventricular artery (AIA) (Table 7).

Table 7. Great cardiac vein and anterior interventricular vein and their variations (mostly own material)

Frequency	100%
Entering the CS	99%
Terminal S-shaped course	32%
Myocardial belt(s) along terminal portion	6%
Intramural course	2%
Aberrant course	1%
Duplication (Pejkovic and Bogdanovic 1992)	3%
Cross-sectional area of terminal part (Hood 1968)	15 (7–37) mm^2
Diameter (anterior interventricular) (Ortale et al. 2001)	2.7 mm (0.9–4.4 mm)
Diameter (great cardiac) (Ortale et al. 2001)	3.9 mm (1.2–6.3 mm)
Diameter (great cardiac) (Pejkovic and Bogdanovic 1992)	5.2 mm (3–7 mm)
Crossing over the stem or all of the branches of the left main coronary artery	49%
Running underneath the diagonal branch	9%
Running underneath circumflex branch	21%
Running underneath both branches	20%

6.4
S-Shaped (Sigmoid) Course of the Great Cardiac Vein

In one-third of our cases, the terminal portion of the GCV ran in an S-shaped course out of the coronary sulcus to the posterolateral wall of the LA, where it emptied into the CS (von Lüdinghausen and Schott 1990) (Figs. 3c, 5a,b).

6.5
Intramyocardial Course of, or Myocardial Bridge Over, the Subepicardial Veins

Intramyocardial courses of the AIV, PIV, and LMV, or myocardial bridges over the veins have been found in 2% of cases examined by von Lüdinghausen and Schott (1990), in 3% by Ortale et al. (2001), and in 5% by Maric et al. (1996). The length of an intramyocardial course was found to range from 2 to 10 mm.

In the heart of the pig, numerous veins are covered by muscular bridges in their subepicardial course; this was observed in 40% of specimens examined by Ratajczyk-Pakalska (1974), and in 21.5% by Berg (1963) (Fig. 17a,b).

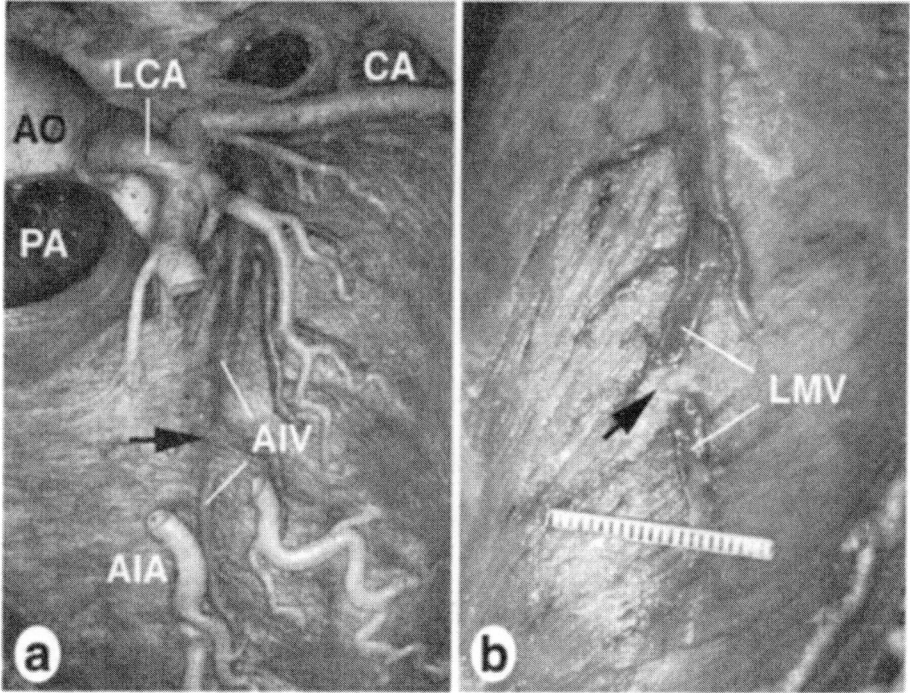

Fig. 17a,b. Intramural courses of, or myocardial bridges over, the great cardiac veins in cadaveric human heart specimens. a Anterior aspect of the heart showing a short intramural course of the AIV (marked by an *arrow*) in the upper third of the anterior interventricular sulcus. b Lateral aspect of the LV showing a short intramural course of the left marginal vein (*arrow*)

6.6
Aberrant Course of the Anterior Interventricular Part of the Great Cardiac Vein

A rarely encountered aberrant course of the AIV was found during the examination of the corrosion casts (von Lüdinghausen and Lechleuthner 1988). Originating at the mid-point along the length of the anterior IV sulcus, it turned to the right, coursed past the conus arteriosus, reached and crossed the right coronary sulcus as one of the ACV, and emptied into the RA. This behavior indicates that the AIV is neither a branch of the GCV nor a tributary of the CS (see Sect. 6.15 "The Anterior Cardiac Veins").

Such an atypical variant can be explained phylogenetically as the result of an unusual development of the ACVs system (Lechleuthner 1987).

Comparative anatomy reveals large ACVs and anterior conus veins, which drain the right lateral and anterior wall of the heart and empty into the RA or the SVC, in some birds and mammalia (Heine 1976). In domestic and wild pigs (Sus scrofa) and in the roe deer (cervus capreolus), the AIV often runs upwards to the transverse sinus between the left auricle and aortic root and finally joins with the azygos vein or directly with the RA (Waldmeier 1928; Gschwend 1931).

In the hearts of hens (Gallus domesticus), the myocardium of the anterior IV groove is often drained by a few enlarged ACVs (Lindsay 1967; Heine 1976; King and McLelland 1978). In these cases the vein which corresponds to the GCV is hypoplastic. Additionally, the vein in question may be interpreted as a remnant of the primitive right coronary vein of reptiles (Grant and Regnier 1926).

In such a case only small veins of the lateral and the posterior walls of the LV drain into the CS. The AIV manifests itself as an enlarged and prolonged conal vein which belongs to the group of ACVs; from an origin in the anterior IV sulcus, it follows a course past the arterial conus and empties directly into the RA (von Lüdinghausen and Schott 1990) (Fig. 18a,b).

6.7
The Ostial (Terminal) Valve of the Great Cardiac Vein

In most of the cases studied, the ostial (terminal) valve of the GCV was situated opposite the entrance of the OV into the initial part of the CS. In 87% (in 91% of cases examined by Pejkovic and Bogdanovic 1992) of the cases studied the valve appeared remarkably developed. Of these, this valve occurred as a membranous leaflet half or three quarters of a circle in shape in 68%. Therefore, it may be designated a unicuspid and functionally insufficient valve. In the remaining 31% there was a bicuspid, and in 1% a tricuspid valve; these are also held to be insufficient because the insertions of the cusps were 1 or 2 mm apart. In 12%–13% of the cases the ostial valve was absent (von Lüdinghausen and Schott 1990; see also Maros et al. 1983; Silver and Rowley 1988) (Fig. 19a–d; Table 8).

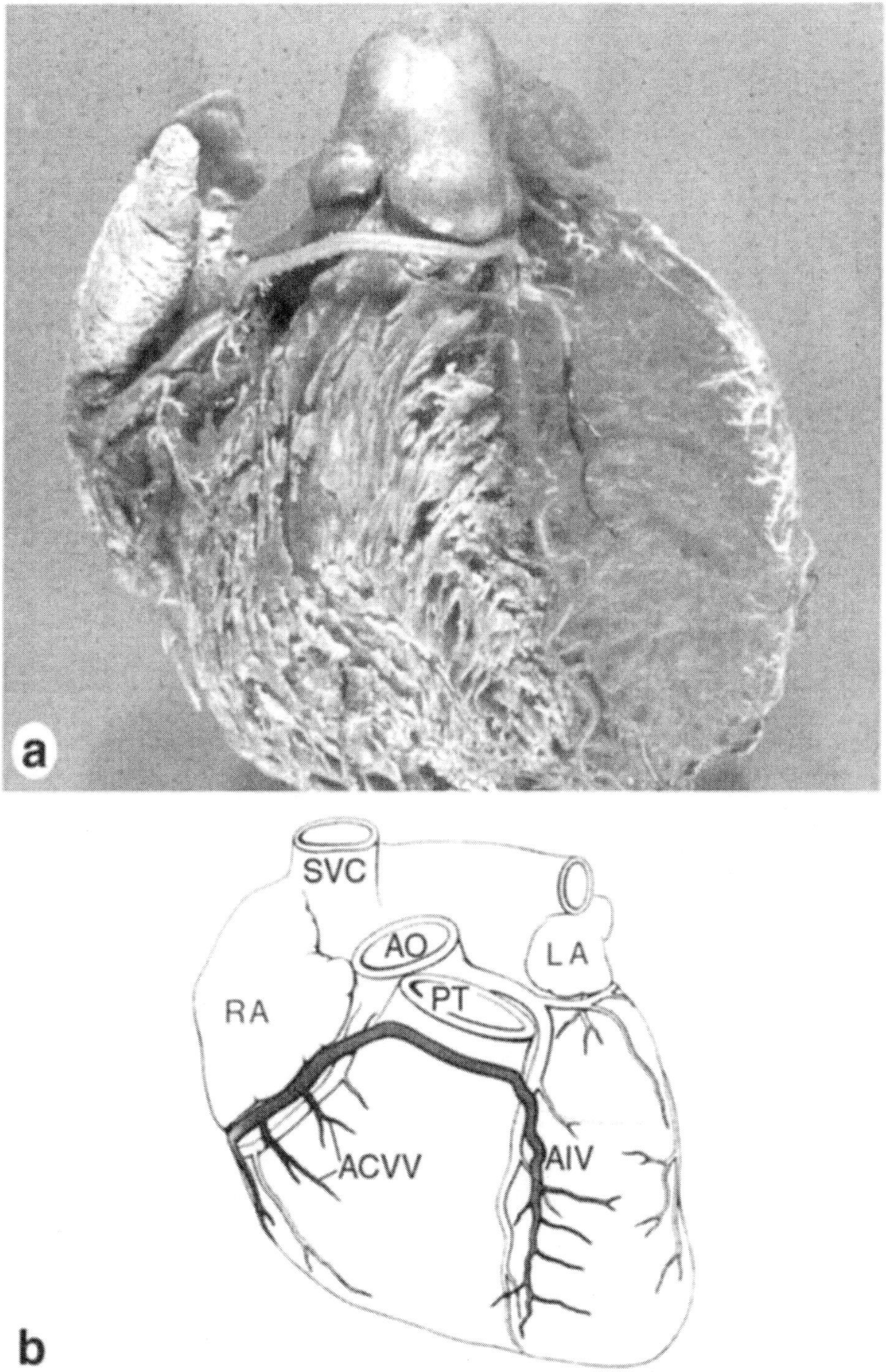

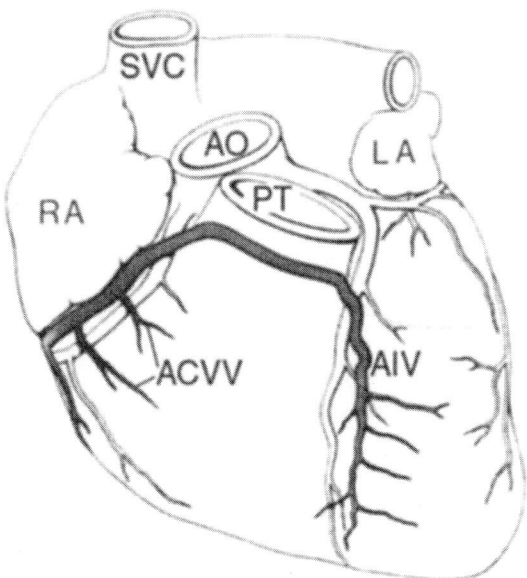

Fig. 18a,b. Anterior aspect of the heart exhibiting an aberrant course of the AIV. The vein originates in the distal anterior IV sulcus, and after leaving it and continuing in a direction towards the right, passes over the arterial conus and the root of the PT. The vein finally joins the ACVs and empties into the RA. Such a vessel may be designated an enlarged ACV or vena conica. a Corrosion specimen. b Schematic drawing

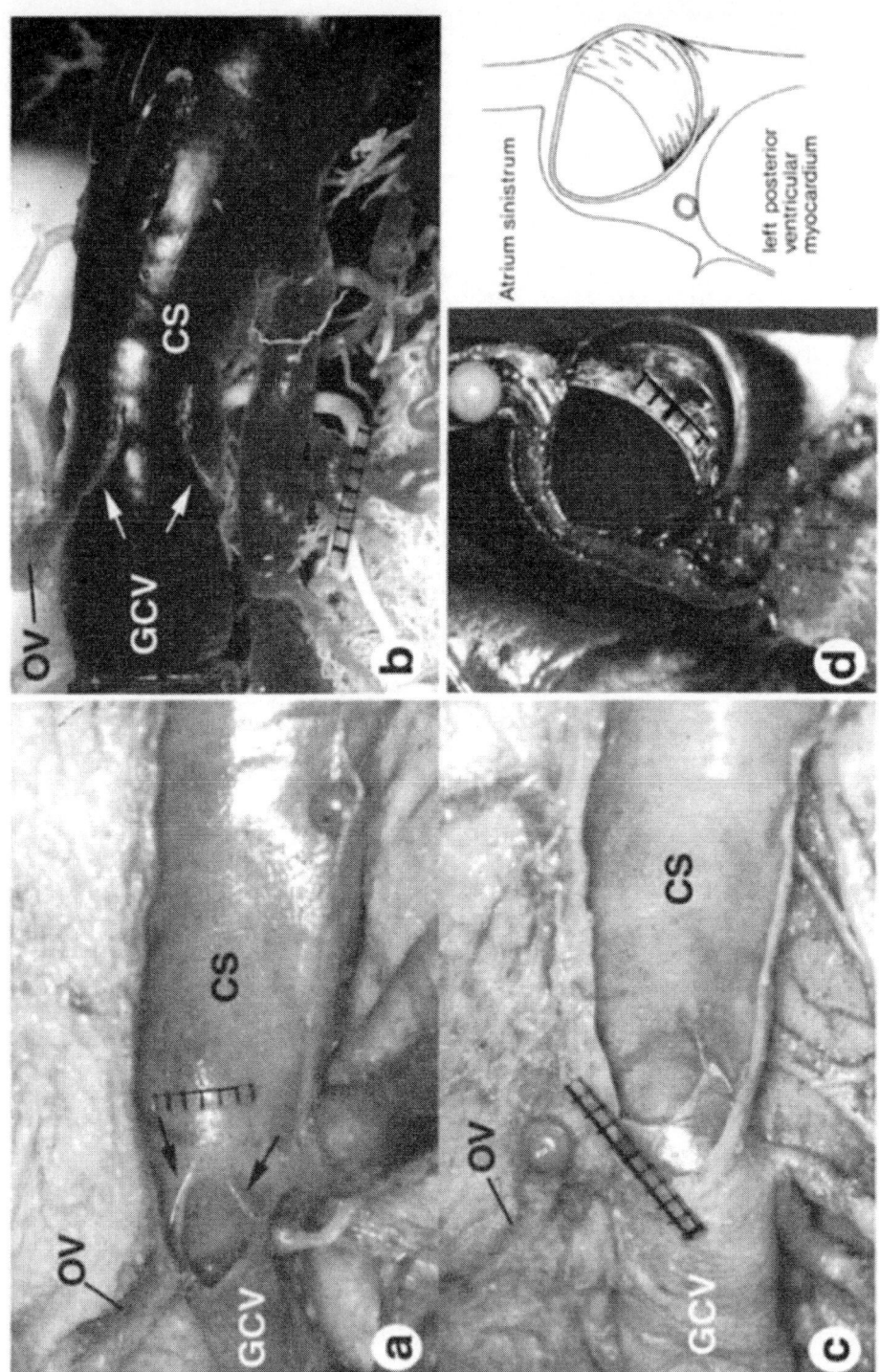

Fig. 19a–d.

Table 8. Shape and incidence of the ostial valve of the GCV

Frequency (own material)	87%
(Pejkovic and Bogdanovic 1992)	91%
(Sarrazin 1965)	75%
Unicuspid valve (own material)	62%
(Mochizuki 1933)	32%
Bicuspid valve (own material)	25%
(Mochzuki 1933)	8%
(Sarrazin 1965)	6%
Tricuspid valve (own material)	1%
Valveless orifice (own material)	13%
(Mochizuki 1933)	25%
(Maros et al. 1983)	13%
(Silver and Rowley 1988)	12%
(Sarrazin 1965)	25%

6.8
The Oblique Vein of the Left Atrium

The OV was present in 84% of our cases (in 97% of those examined by Parsonnet 1953, in 92% by Maric et al. 1996, and in 43% by Ortale et al. 2001); it was 2–3 cm in length and 0.4–1.8 mm in diameter (average diameter 1.0 mm). It traversed and descended the left lateral and posterior wall of the LA and entered the CS at its left end, i.e., 1–12 mm distal to, and to the right of, the terminal valve of GCV (Table 9).

Table 9. Oblique vein of the left atrium (mostly own material)

Incidence	84%
Diameter (Ortale et al. 2001)	1.0 mm (0.4–1.8 mm)
Length	2–3 cm
Completely regressed to a fibrous cord	12%
Not exactly verifiable	3%–4%
Persistent left superior vena cava	0.5%

Fig. 19a–d. Ostial valves of the GCV and their various forms. a A CS opened to show a bicuspid form of the terminal valve of the GCV (marked by *black arrows*) which, because the valvular insertions are not close together, appears insufficient. **b** Corrosion cast of a CS. The impressions made by two endothelial folds corresponding to a bicuspid valve (marked by *white arrows*) are visible at the junction of the GCV and the CS. **c** A CS opened to show a unicuspid form of the (obviously insufficient) terminal valve of the GCV (marked by a *millimeter scale*). **d** Photograph of a unicuspid valve (different from that shown in c) (marked by a *millimeter scale*) and corresponding drawing

In 12% the vein was replaced by a tiny cord or string of connective tissue attached to the left end of the CS. Given the reliability of its existence as a vein or string, we are able to recommend it as a relatively safe landmark (as an "operative guide" according to Parsonnet 1953) designating the beginning of the CS (see Chap. 5.6"The Proximal Origin of the CS and Its Landmarks").

The entrance of the OV into the CS was marked by a small endothelial fold or by a functionally sufficient or insufficient pair of semilunar ostial valves. Tandler (1926), however, did not observe ostial valves at the opening of the OV into the CS.

The angle between the axis of the OV and the CS varied between 25° and 50°.

The OV constitutes the remnant of either the embryologically important left sinus horn or the superior cardinal vein. It has also been designated as a vestige of the left SVC (Vlodaver et al 1976; Langman 1977; Anderson and Becker 1982; Moore 1988). The left SVC is persisting in various mammalian species like rabbits and pigs (according to the findings of Grant and Regnier 1926). In rare cases, the left SVC (Cuvieri's duct) persists in some patients who are symptomless when there is an open communication between the left subclavian vein and the CS (Schütz 1914; von Lüdinghausen and Lechleuthner 1988) (Figs. 3a,b, 6a,c, 11a, 12a,b).

6.9
The Posterior Interventricular Vein

The PIV was seen to exist in all heart specimens studied by Parsonnet (1953), von Lüdinghausen (1987), Maric et al. (1996), and Ortale et al. (2001). In 75% of the cases of von Lüdinghausen (1987) and of Waller and Schlant (1994) the vein arose as a single vessel and in 24% as two vessels, sometimes almost equally formed, from the superficial venous network at the cardiac apex, ascending in the posterior IV sulcus to the crux cordis to drain the CS or – rarely – the RA directly (Figs. 3a–c, 4, 11d, 14, 16c, 20a,b, 21a,b).

The two veins incorporated the posterior IV branch of the right (or occasionally the left) circumflex branch of the left coronary artery and joined together in the upper third of the posterior IV sulcus.

The vein and its tributaries drained the posterior "diaphragmatic" walls of both the RA and LV as well as the apical area; by means of its septal venous channels it drained the posterior third or two thirds of the IV septum. In all our specimens the posterior intramural (perforating) channels left the myocardium, formed posterior septal veins of 1–2 mm length and ran at almost right angles to the PIV (Parsonnet 1953).

In 81% of the cases studied, the terminal portion (12–28 mm in length) of the PIV turned at an obtuse angle to the left, and after following an oblique course emptied into the terminal CS adjacent to its atrial ostium (90%) or into the RA (2.5%).

In 19% of the cases studied, both the entire PIV and posterior IV sulcus followed the same straight course.

The stem of the PIV exhibited a diameter ranging between 2.1 and 5.3 mm, with an average of 3.6 mm (also according to Ortale et al. 2001).

The ostium was marked by a variably formed unicuspid valve (50%) or bicuspid valve (11%). In 39% of our cases, no valve was evident (see Sect. 6.17 "The Ostial Valves of the Cardiac Veins").

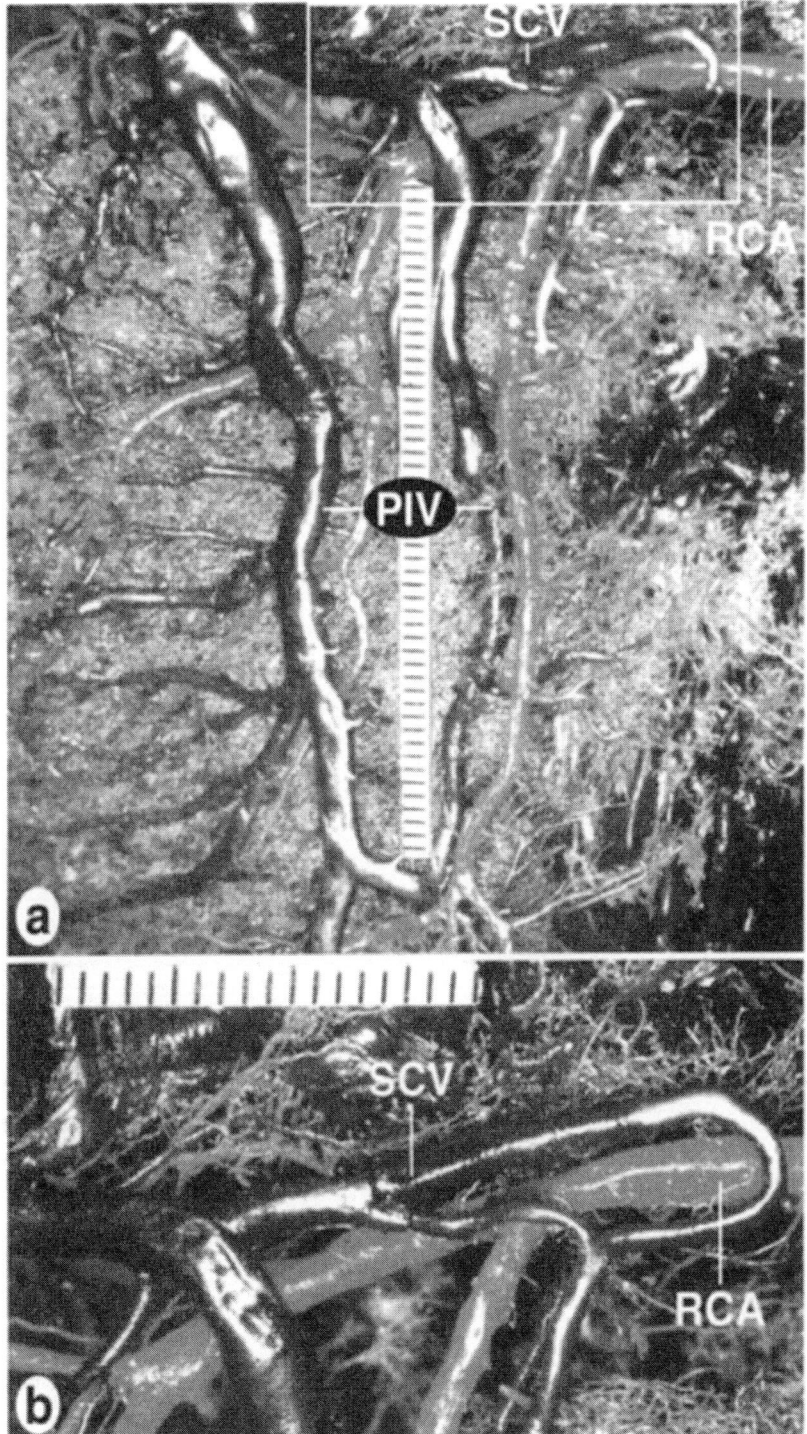

Fig. 20a,b. Corrosion cast of a human heart specimen showing the diaphragmatic surface. a There is a duplication of both the PIV and the SCV. b Duplication of the SCV. The two veins are interconnected (shown in magnification from the *rectangle* in a)

Table 10. Posterior interventricular vein; frequency, terminal portion, mode of opening, and ostial valves (mostly own material)

Frequency	Single	75%
	Double (two vessels)	24%
	Triple (three vessels)	0.5%
Terminal portion	Straight course	19%
	Moderate angulation	46%
	Severe angulation	35%
	Bulbous dilation	19%
	Myocardial cover	2.5%
	Sinus coronarius "duplex"	1%
Opening	Into the CS	90%
	Into the right atrium	2.5%
	Between the leaflets of the valve of the CS	0.5%
	Not determined in cases without a valve of the CS	8%
Diameter of the terminal part (Ortale et al. 2001)		3.6 mm (2.1–5.3 mm)
Mean cross-sectional area at ostial opening (Hood 1968)		6–25 mm^2 (13 mm^2)
Ostial valve of the PIV	Frequency in all hearts (Parsonnet 1953)	87%
	Unicuspid	50%
	Bicuspid	11%
	Ectopic (uni- or bicuspid) valve	19%
	Missing valve	39%

In 19% of the cases, the terminal part of the middle cardiac vein was bulbous in form, due to the presence of an ectopic valve which occluded the vein at a distance of 10 mm from the CS. Thus, the terminal part of the vein was integrated into the space of the CS. When compared with the AIV, the PIV is the stronger vessel (Table 10).

6.9.1
Ostial Valves

In one-third of our cases the ostia of the posterior septal veins or intramural channels exhibited numerous uni- or bicuspid ostial valves ("Astklappen") (Fig. 21a,b).

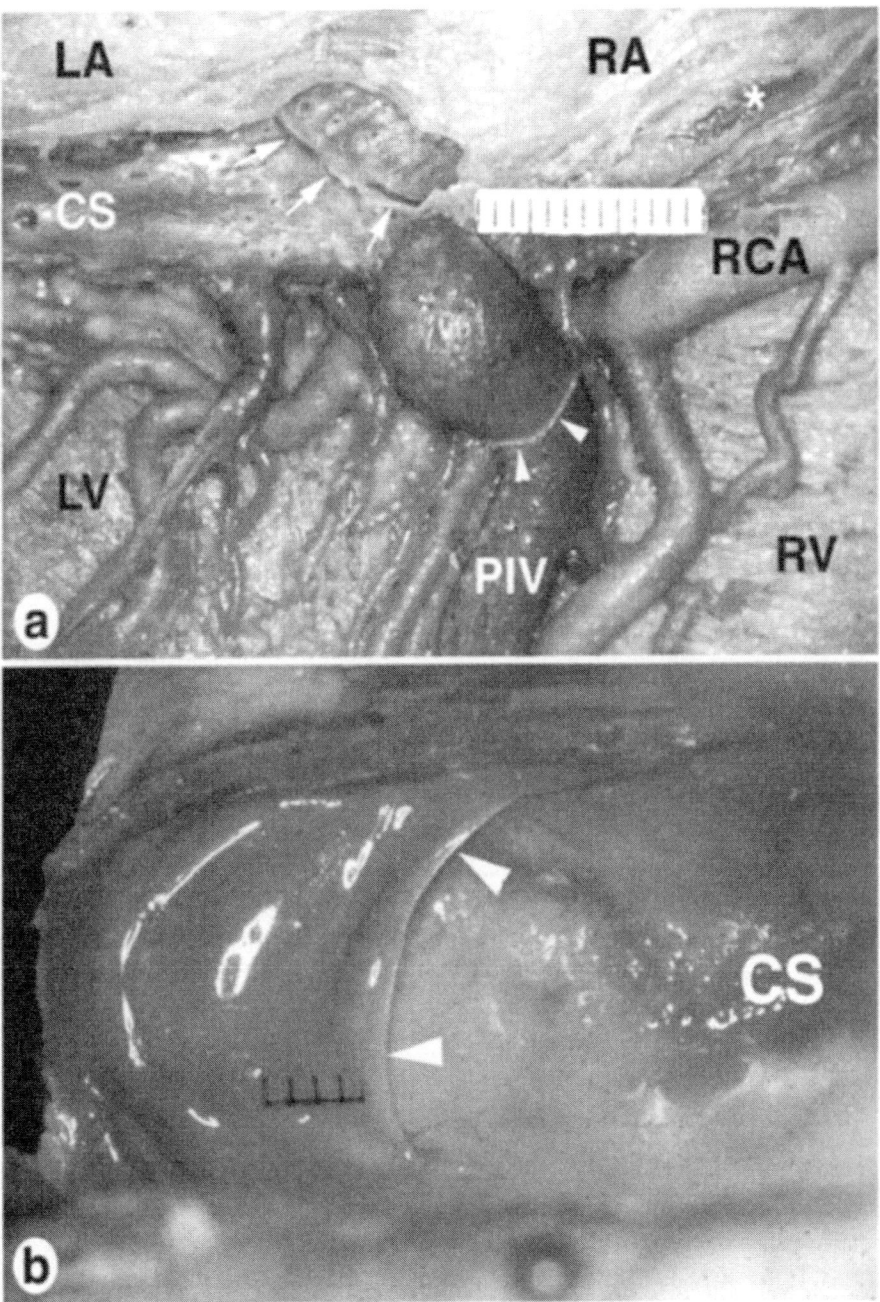

Fig. 21a,b. Ostial valve of the PIV. a An injected cadaveric specimen showing a unicuspid ostial valve of the PIV (indicated by *arrowheads*) at the junction of its straight and oblique sections; the oblique part of the PIV is integrated into the CS. b A complete (obviously sufficient) ostial valve of the PIV (marked by *arrowheads*) in the opened terminal segment of a CS, as seen from superior

Peculiarities

In 2.5% of the cases studied the terminal portion of the PIV was wrapped in a myocardial coat (see Chap. 5.4 "Isolated Myocardial Belts in the Terminal Portions of Other Cardiac Veins").

In one case the vein emptied into the terminal CS between the leaflets of the ostial valve. The opening of the vein could not exactly be determined in cases where no valve of the CS existed (8%).

In one of our cases there was a triple version of the PIV in the apical part of the posterior IV sulcus.

In another case the terminal oblique part of the PIV was widened and covered by a myocardial coat in the same way as the CS itself. This anomaly was designated a sinus coronarius duplex or accessory CS (von Lüdinghausen et al. 1994) (see Chap. 4.10 "Duplication of the CS").

6.10
The Septal Veins

Along its course, the AIV receives three types of short branches. These are (from the right) small veins draining the anterior walls of the RV, (from the left) small veins draining the lateral wall of the LV (Tandler 1913, Bargmann 1963), and anterior (perforating) septal veins collecting numerous smaller and larger intramural venous channels.

In most cases it is possible to distinguish between anterior and posterior SVs which empty into the AIV and PIV, respectively. With regard to the venous drainage of the IV septum, four irregularly terminated territories may be differentiated: anterior, posterior, right superior, and left superior (Parsonnet 1953; McAlpine 1975; von Lüdinghausen 1987).

The subendocardial layers of the IV septum are characterized by numerous well-developed smallest cardiac vessels (Moir et al. 1963; Shiki et al. 1986) (Figs. 22a–c, 23a,b).

6.10.1
Anterior and Posterior Territories
of the Interventricular Septum

The anterior and posterior territories may be divided into right and left halves and their related right and left anterior septal veins and right and left posterior septal veins. This pattern corresponds to the finding of a duplicate (right and left) AIV and a duplicate (right and left) PIV in the anterior and posterior IV sulcus, respectively. A long duplication of the AIV (of more than 3 cm length) was observed in 3% and of the PIV in 24% of our cases.

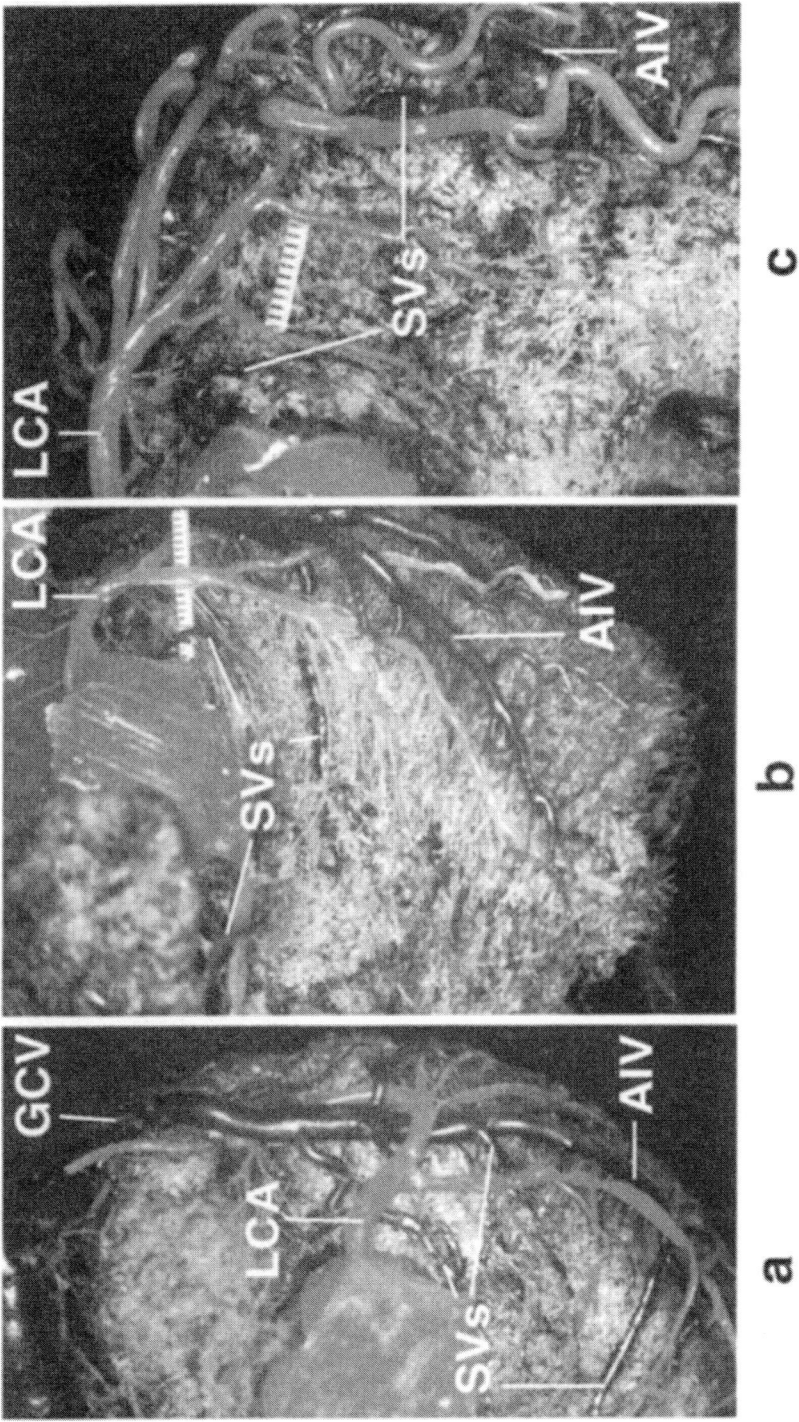

Fig. 22a–c. Venous drainage of the superior and anterior parts of the interventricular septum as seen in corrosion casts. **a, c** Superior and anterior septal veins (SVs) course beneath the main stem of the LCA and the AIA and empty into the AIV. **b** The right superior SV courses to the right coronary sulcus and opens into the RA; the left superior and anterior septal SVs course to the anterior IV sulcus and empty into the AIV

6.10.2
Left Superior Septal Vein

The largest and longest intramural venous channel (almost 2–3 mm in diameter) in the IV septum was the LSSV; it was found to drain the myocardium of the crista supraventricularis in about 55% of our cases. The vessel coursed in the subendocardial layers of the right outflow area and collected frequent small veins of the superior third of the IV septum before emptying into the distal AIV. Numerous small, secondary veins reached the large primary vein, opening at a right angle into it. The course of this LSSV corresponds almost exactly with that of the left superior septal artery. (Fig. 22 a,c).

6.10.3
Anterior Septal Veins

Another large anterior septal venous channel (but a smaller one than that previously described) was found to drain the middle third of the IV septum and also open into the AIV.

This vessel occurred in about 35% of our cases and its course corresponded approximately with that of the left descending artery (moderator band artery). In the anterior half of the IV septum, numerous small SVs proceeded in our cases in an anterior direction to reach the AIV, and the veins of the posterior half of the IV septum in a posterior direction to empty into the PIV. (Fig. 22 b).

6.10.4
Right Superior Septal Vein

A third large vein was seen to drain the right superior third of the IV septum and crista supraventricularis in 28% of our cases. This vessel was designated the RSSV; it drained the myocardium beneath the stem of the right coronary artery and joined the anterior cardiac veins and their intramural venous sinus before it opened into the RA. When the anterior and posterior channels reached the surface of the myocardium in the anterior and posterior IV sulcus, they formed in our cases short venous trunks of 1–2 mm length which emptied into the AIV or PIV. (Fig. 22 b).

6.10.5
Venous Valves (Astklappen)

In one-third of our cases, posterior SVs exhibited frequent uni- or bicuspid ostial valves (see the previous chapter). The anterior SVs showed only few unicuspid and incomplete ostial valves (Fig. 23a,b).

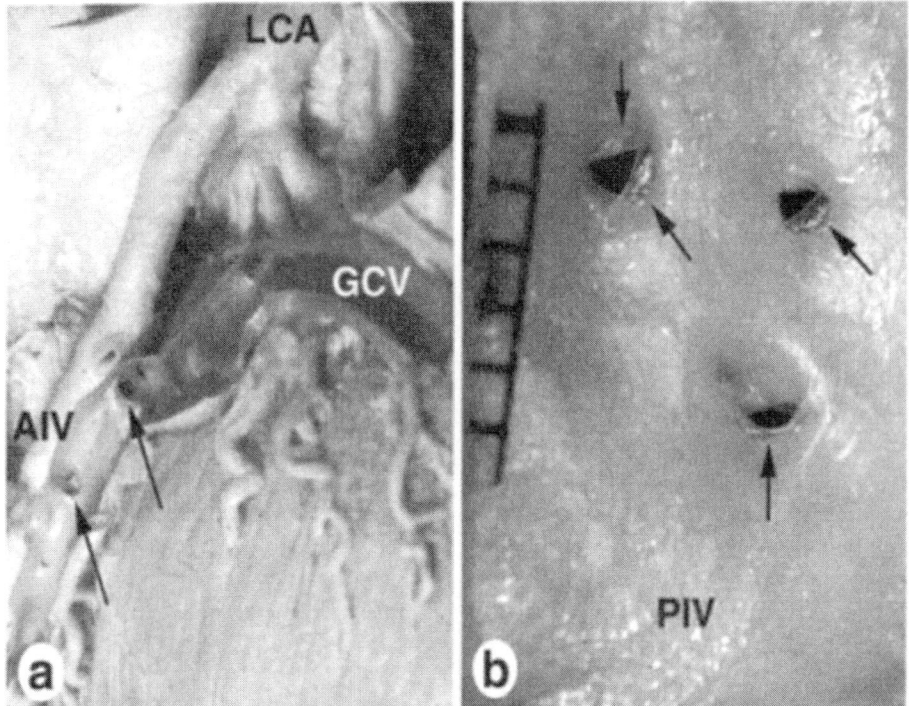

Fig. 23a,b. Ostial valves ("Astklappen") of the left superior, anterior, and posterior septal veins. a AIV opened to show incomplete unicuspid ostial valves of the left superior and anterior septal veins (marked by *black arrows*). b PIV opened to show incomplete uni- and bicuspid valves of the posterior septal veins (marked by *black arrows*)

6.10.6
Venous Drainage of the AV Junction

At the AV junction there are frequent irregular and thin-walled venous channels and sinusoids which are intimately related to the AV node and common bundle tissue. The larger venous channels possess all the histological features of thin-walled veins, whereas the sinusoids consist of nothing more than a single layer of endothelial cells. The vessels communicate with, and drain directly into, the RA or the CS (Truex and Schwartz 1951; von Lüdinghausen et al. 1995).

6.11
The Posterior Vein(s) of the Left Ventricle

The PVLV existed as a single large vessel in 63% of the cases studied by Parsonnet (1953) and in our material. Instead of a single strong vessel, there was a group of duplicate developed, medium-sized vessels and multiple small vessels veins in 33% of our specimens. Altogether, PVsLV were seen in 99% of our specimens and in 95% of the cases studied by Ortale et al. (2001). The diameter ranged from 1.0–5.5 mm, with an average of 2.4 mm.

Table 11. Frequency and mode of opening of the posterior vein of the left ventricle (mostly own material)

Frequency	99%
Diameter (Ortale et al. 2001)	2.4 mm (1.0–55.5 mm)
Single, developed, strong vessel	63%
Duplicate developed, medium-sized veins	23%
Multiple (3–5) small vessels	9%
No posterior ventricular but strong left marginal vein	5%
Mode of opening	
Into the CS with ostial valve (Parsonnet 1953)	37%
Into the CS with ostial valve (Maros et al. 1983)	77%
5–15 mm distal to the ostial valve	57%
15–25 mm distal to the ostial valve	17%
25–35 mm distal to the ostial valve	8%
35–45 mm distal to the ostial valve	5%
Into the great cardiac vein without ostial valve	13%
Terminal bulb	5%
Myocardial belts of the terminal portion	2%

The vein(s) drained the lateral and posterior wall of the left ventricle. As a rule, in our cases the single PVLV or multiple PVsLV opened into the proximal second- and third-centimeter segment of the CS, or led – in a few instances 196 into the terminal portion of the GCV (von Lüdinghausen 1987); in a few cases there was no PVLV in existence but a strong LMV draining the posterior wall of the LV (Table 11).

In most cases the PVLV was not accompanied by the corresponding artery (posterior branch of the LV); on the contrary, the latter crossed the vein at a right angle, at the mid-point along its length (Fig. 3a–c, 4).

Also, in most cases the PVLV features a sufficient valve at its opening (5–25 mm proximal to the atrial valve of the CS) (see also Sect. 6.17 "The Ostial Valves of the Cardiac Veins").

When the vein empties into the CS near to the atrial ostium, its retrograde perfusion is rendered difficult or impossible.

6.12
The Small Cardiac Vein

The SCV is a minute tributary of the CS; it originates in the posterior part of the right coronary sulcus and runs along the base of the right ventricle, sometimes receiving the right marginal vein. The SCV was a vessel worthy of mention in 29% of our

Table 12. Small cardiac vein; frequency, mode of opening, and size (mostly own material)

Frequency (1 mm or more in diameter)	29%
Frequency (less than 1 mm in diameter)	40%
Absent or fibrous cord	31%
Opening	
Into the posterior interventricular vein	96%
Into the CS	4.0%
Mean cross-sectional area (Hood 1968)	1.0 mm^2
Terminal anastomosing loop	4.0%
Absent	36%

specimens, in 37% of the cases studied by Parsonnet (1953), and in 54% of the cases studied by Ortale et al. (2001). It was given consideration only when it exhibited a diameter of approximately 1.0 mm or more. In the other cases, the diameter of the SCV was less than 1 mm, or the vein was thread-like or just non-existent (von Lüdinghausen 1987).

According to its caliber, the SCV drains a minor or larger district of the posterior and lateral wall of the right ventricle. It runs parallel (above or below) to the right coronary artery in the right coronary sulcus and empties into the PIV or directly into the CS.

In one-third of cases (von Lüdinghausen 1987) the SCV was reduced to a fibrous cord or thread (Table 12). According to the investigations of Parsonnet (1953), in three out of seven cases in which a SCV was present, there was also a subendocardial, intramural, or subepicardial venous sinus. This argues against the designation of these veins and sinuses as identical (see Sect. 6.16 "The Venous Drainage of the Papillary Muscles") (Fig. 4, 14, 20a,b).

Peculiarities

In 10% of the cases studied by Mechanik (1934) and Aho (1950) the SCV was the continuation of the RMV.

In some cases the SCV has been found to drain the RMV and a few of the ACVs. In two corrosion specimens, there was a duplication of the SCV: the two vessels fused at 25 mm along their length, forming a (terminal anastomosing) venous loop.

6.13
The Left Marginal Vein

The LMV was present in 88% of the specimens we studied (in 73% of cases examined by Parsonnet 1953, in 80% by Pejkovic and Bogdanovic 1992, with a diameter varying from 1 to 3 mm and an average of 2.24 mm, and in 97% by Ortale et al. 2001, with a diameter varying from 0.8–4.5 mm and an average of 2.3 mm).

The LMV emptied into the GCV in 79% and into the CS in 21% of the cases studied (81% and 19%, respectively, in cases examined by Ortale et al. (2001) and 88% and 12%, respectively, by Pejkovic and Bogdanovic (1992) (see also Sect. 6.17 "The Ostial Valves of the Cardiac Veins") (Figs. 3a, 17).

6.14
The Right Marginal Vein

The RMV is a vessel of varying length and caliber. It was found in 13% of the hearts studied by Parsonnet (1953), in 82% of those studied by Mierzwa and Kozielec (1975), in 87% of the cases studied by von Lüdinghausen (1987), and in 92% of cases studied by Ortale et al. (2001).

In cases in which there is an "early" origin of the RMV, some authors tend to count the RMV among the ACVs. This may explain the great variability of percentages regarding the occurrence of the RMV.

The initial branches originated from the cardiac apex. The main trunk ascended along the right border of the right ventricle from the apex, subepicardially and in adipose tissue, receiving as tributaries small venous branches from the posterior and anterior surfaces of the right ventricle (Mierzwa and Kozielec 1975).

The diameter of the main trunk ranged from 0.5 to 2.9 mm, with an average of 1.8 mm according to Ortale et al. (2001).

In 33% of the cases studied by Mierzwa and Kozielec (1975) and von Lüdinghausen (1987), the RMV continued in the posterior part of the right coronary sulcus as the SCV; in a further 33% it joined the group of the ACVs (without having developed into the SCV) and emptied directly into the right auricle or into a venous sinus of the RA (see Chap. 7.2 "The Veins of the Right Atrium").

6.15
The Anterior Cardiac Veins

The ACVs – including the right lateral marginal and conus veins – were present in 92% of cases examined by Esperanca Pina (1975) and von Lüdinghausen (1987),and 91% of cases examined by Ortale and Marquez (1998). The ACVs are variable in number, extension, and caliber. They originate in the anterior surface of the RV and run almost parallel to the right margin and the RMV (Esperanca Pina 1975). According to the findings of Parsonnet (1953) and McAlpine (1975), the ACVs receive blood from the right two-thirds of the myocardium of the anterior and anterolateral walls of the RV.

The ACVs exhibited various distribution patterns:
1. In about 28% of the cases we studied, the ACVs reached the right atrial wall – a little above the right coronary sulcus – as single vessels and emptied directly into the RA.
2. In 6% of our cases, most ACVs joined together and formed a venous trunk of 2 to 5 mm length, which approached the epicardial surface of the right atrial wall.

3. In 66% of our cases, single anterior veins or their venous stems did not terminate directly in the RA but emptied beforehand into a venous sinus in the anterior wall of the right auricle (Mochizuki 1933; von Lüdinghausen 1987; Ortale and Marquez 1998) (see next paragraph).

In one-third of our cases the RMV joins the group of the ACVs (without having developed into the SCV), and in several cases the conus vein and the vein draining the soft tissue between the aortic bulb and the PT also belonged to the group of the ACVs. In a few cases, an anterior cardiac vein joined with the RMV, proceeded as the SCV in the right coronary sulcus, and emptied into the posterior IV vein.

One anterior cardiac vein (of more than 1 mm in diameter) was found in 24%, two veins (of more than 1 mm diameter) in 48%, and three veins (of more than 1 mm diameter) in 28% of our cases. Numerous additional thin and thread-like veins had developed in between the larger ACVs. Ortale and Marquez (1998) found up to 15 smaller or larger veins after meticulous dissection of the anterior cardiac wall.

In 87% of the cases studied by Parsonnet (1953), the ACVs exhibited significant anastomotic channels with the major tributaries of the CS (Figs. 24a,b).

Peculiarities

1. In rare cases reported by McAlpine (1975), an extremely thick conus vein had developed from a dense venous network embracing the conus arteriosus and the bulb of the aorta. The vein was also noted by Mierzwa and Kozielec (1975) and seen to cross the pulmonary conus and empty – together with other anterior veins – into the right auricle.
2. One of our specimens exhibited a unique long, strong ACV which was the continuation of an aberrant AIV. This vein has already been described in detail (see Sect. 6.6 "Aberrant Course of the Anterior Interventricular Part of the Great Cardiac Vein").

According to Mierzwa and Kozielec (1975) the atrioventricular veins were numerous, very variable and very small slender vessels situated deep in the right coronary sulcus next to the annulus fibrosus of the TRI, collecting blood from the anterior and lateral external surface of the right annulus fibrosus and emptying into some of the venous sinuses of the RA (according to Mierzwa and Kozielec 1975).

In summary, the ACVs are the chief instrument of venous drainage of the RV (Smith 1962).

6.16
The Venous Drainage of the Papillary Muscles

The papillary muscles are drained by one to three veins of an arboriform type (according to Ratajczyk-Pakalska et al. 1990). These vessels originate on the endocardium and run towards the larger subepicardially situated veins. According to Unger (1938), the right papillary muscles are completely drained by vessels of the SCVS. The left papillary muscles are drained by veins of both the GCVS and SCVS (Unger 1938; Rosinia and Low 1986).

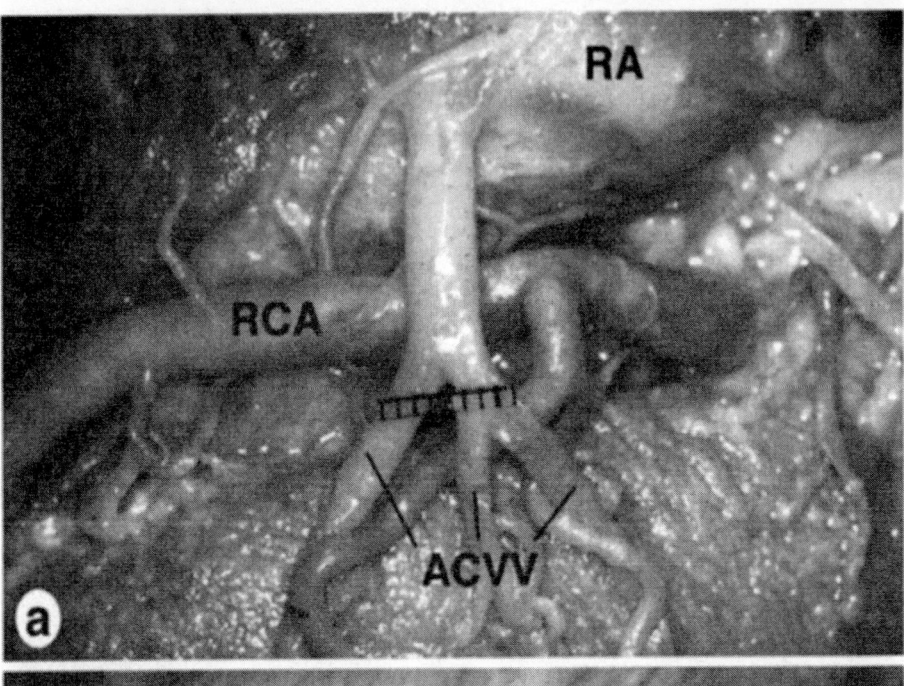

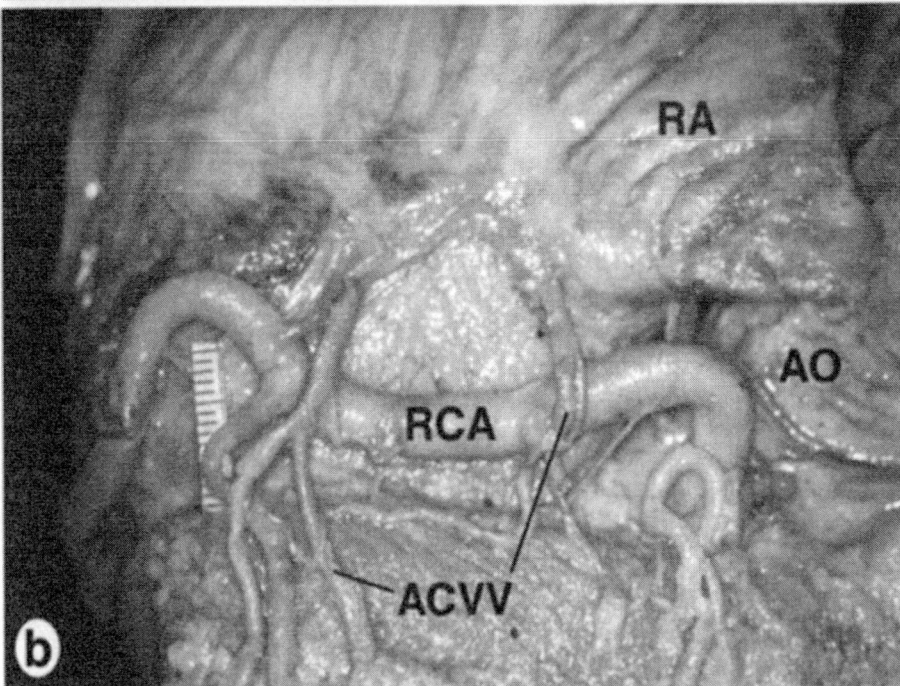

Fig. 24a,b. Anterior surface of the right atrium and right coronary sulcus of cadaveric specimens showing the mode of distribution of the ACVs. a Three ACVs join together and form a common stem which passes over the RCA and empties into the RA. b The ACV form two common stems which empty into the RA

6.17
The Ostial Valves of Cardiac Veins

Where the smaller cardiac veins (those with a diameter less than 1.5 mm) enter the main cardiac venous stems at an oblique angle, there were almost incomplete and obviously insufficient unicuspid ostial valves ("Astklappen") in 31% of the cases studied. In a few cases such "Astklappen" were found at the openings of the septal branches into the PIV. However, the openings of the vv cardiacae into the CS (namely the GCV with its ostial valve, the LMV, the PVLV, and the PIV) were found to have completely closing (in 28.5% of the cases), or incompletely closing (in 26%), unicuspid and bicuspid valves ("Mündungsklappen" according to Staubesand and Rulffs 1958). In about 45% of our cases there were no real valves at the openings of the cardiac veins into the CS. In 12% we found ostial valves at the openings of atrial veins and ACVs.

In some cases we found "recessed" ostial valves of the GCV, LMV, and PIV which were situated 1–5 mm proximal from the related orifice (the term "recessed" was first used by von Kügelgen 1958).

Where comparative anatomy is concerned, the quantity and quality of cardiac venous valves depends on the size of the mammalian heart. Small hearts exhibit only a few venous valves; most of them seem to be rudimentary. According to Staubesand and Rulffs (1958), valvular anomalies in small veins are seen more frequently in tissues of older individuals and are an indication of degeneration and accidental involution. In large animals, such as horses, elephants, and giraffes, cardiac veins with more and stronger venous valves are observed (Lechleuthner 1987). In most cases, the ostial valves have one or two cusps, which – as in human beings – seem mostly to be of an insufficient nature (Figs. 19a–d, 21a,b, 23a,b).

6.18
The Relationships Between Cardiac Veins and Coronary Arteries

Almost all the main ventricular veins appear to have a close relationship with the interventricular and coronary sulci and the right and left cardiac margins, and the arteries of these landmarks.

Thus, the two marginal and two interventricular venous stems were found in the majority of our cases to enjoy close relationships with the marginal and IV arteries in the sense that the veins accompanied the arteries on their courses, often crossing under or over them, or winding around them (Maric et al. 1996). As a consequence, single cases of compression of a major vein by a major artery were observed (von Lüdinghausen 1976, 1987) (Fig. 25a,b).

Peculiarities

The AIV runs adjacent and in very close proximity to the anterior IV branch of the left coronary artery and is partly hidden in the fatty tissue of the anterior IV sulcus.

In 49% of our cases the anterior branch of the GCV accompanied the similarly named arterial branch on its left side, and crossed over the diagonal branch and the

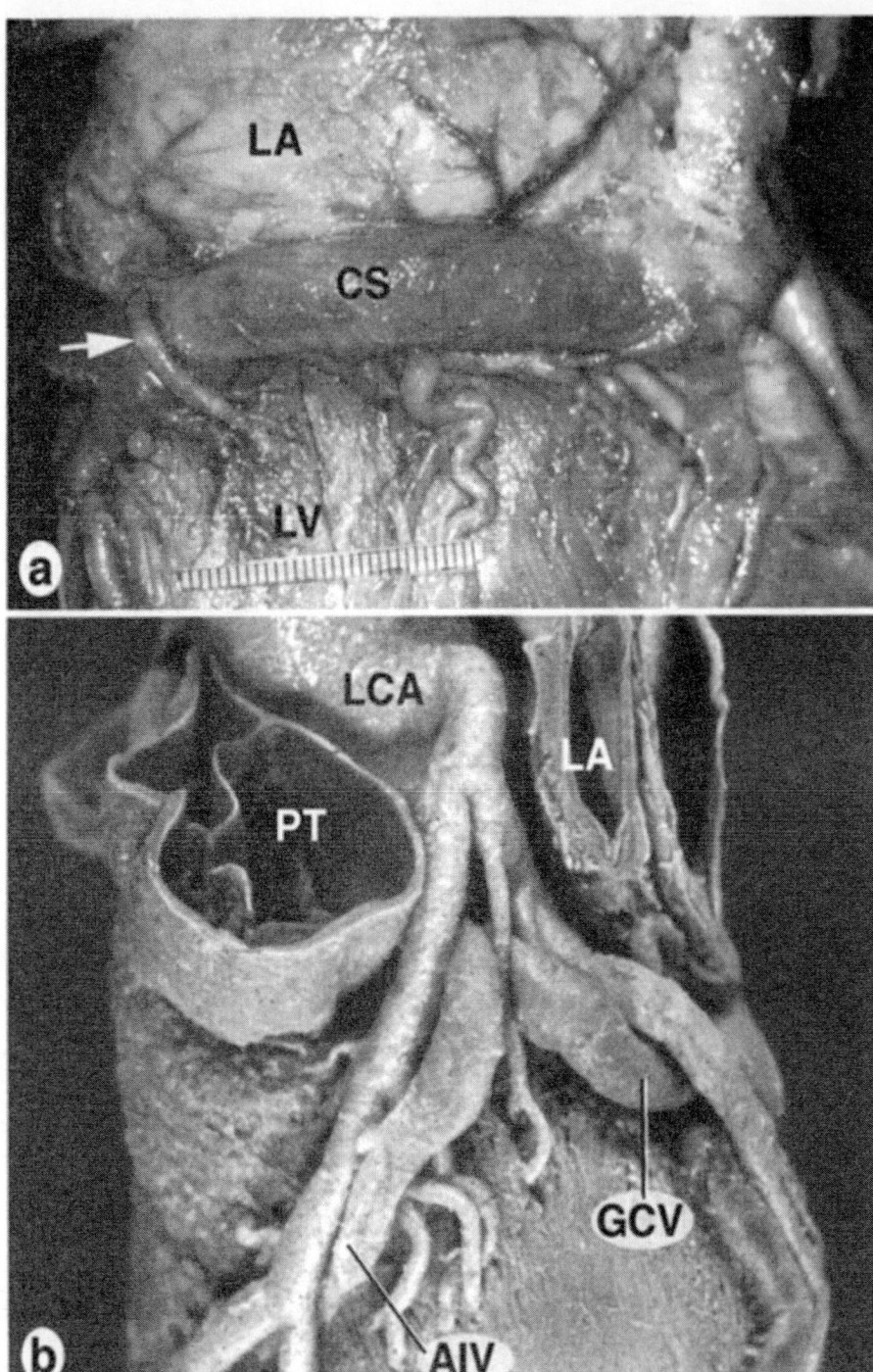

Fig. 25a,b. The relationship between cardiac veins and arterial branches as seen in cadaveric specimens. a The junction of the GCV and CS is surrounded and obviously compressed, or even strangulated, by a branch of the left circumflex artery (marked by a *white arrow*). b The junction of AIV and GCV is compressed and constricted by a diagonal branch of the left coronary artery

circumflex branch of the left coronary artery to reach the left coronary sulcus (von Lüdinghausen 1987).

In 9% of our cases the AIV crossed under the diagonal branch but over the circumflex branch, in 21% it crossed over the diagonal branch but under the circumflex branch, and in 20% it crossed under both the diagonal and circumflex branches.

The PIV in the posterior IV sulcus was accompanied on its course by the posterior IV branch of the right coronary artery (in 10% of the cases the posterior IV branch was a branch of the circumflex branch of the left coronary artery). A duplication of the PIV had developed in the apical part of the posterior IV sulcus in 45% of the cases and the two veins accompanied the terminal part of the corresponding posterior IV branch.

The ACVs coursed directly to the right coronary sulcus. In the majority of our specimens the veins crossed over (in 62% of cases) or under (in 18% of the cases) the right coronary artery (see also McAlpine 1975). In 20% of cases both modes of crossing were observed.

Exceptions

The PVLV and RMV are exceptions here, ramifying almost without arterial attendants (see Sect. 6.11). Given the diversity of the ramification patterns of the arteries, venous distribution patterns are also highly variable (Vlodaver et al. 1976; von Lüdinghausen and Schott 1990).

6.19
The Veins of the Visceral Serosa

In the ventricular subepicardial layers there were numerous smallest capillary networks and drainage veins, apparently draining into the more deeply situated branches of the epimurally distributed veins of the GCVS.

The veins of the visceral serosa of the right and left atrial epicardium traverse the atrial myocardium perpendicularly and empty directly into the corresponding atrium. In view of their shortness and opening pattern, they belong to the SCVS. They could easily be seen with the naked eye in cases of congestion in individuals who had suffered from decompensation following coronary heart disease, left-heart insufficiency, and pulmonary venous congestion. The question of how far these veins contribute to the secretion of serous fluid into the pericardial sac remains unanswered.

6.20
Venous Anastomoses

From a determination of the distribution pattern and the modes of openings of the greater ventricular veins, it emerged that the veins in the IV sulci (AIV and PIV) and at the margins (right and left marginal veins) exhibit a relative consistency of origin, course, and termination, while the veins between these axial venous stems – for example the PVLV and the ACVs – are rather irregular in the number, size, course, mode of opening, and frequency of anastomoses.

In general, there are widespread anastomoses at all levels of cardiac venous circulation, on a scale exceeding that of the arteries, and amounting to a veritable venous plexus according to some authors (Truex and Angulo 1952; Baroldi and Scomazzoni 1965; Williams et al. 1995). Not only are adjacent veins often connected, but connections also exist between tributaries of the CS and those of the ACVs (Mierzwa and Kozielec 1975). The highest density of subepicardial venous anastomoses is found in the apical area of the heart (Lechleuthner and von Lüdinghausen 1986; von Lüdinghausen 1987).

Two large axially orientated circles and one large horizontally orientated venous circle in the coronary sulcus embrace the entire heart (McAlpine 1975; Lechleuthner 1987). These circles consist of:
1. The RMV, the LMV, and atrial veins
2. The AIV and PIV, and atrial veins
3. The CS, GCV, SCV, conus vein, and further intercommunicating veins

In the same way as the ventricular and atrial branches of the coronary arteries, the cardiac veins connect with extracardiac vessels, chiefly the vasa vasorum of the large vessels and mediastinal veins (Williams et al. 1995; von Lüdinghausen et al. 1995). Arteriovenous anastomoses – as described by Ratajczyk-Pakalska (1975) – have not been found macroscopically in our material.

6.21
The Veins of the Vasa Vasorum of the Coronary Arteries, Aorta Ascendens and Pulmonary Trunk

Clarke (1965b) found that the veins of the vasa vasorum of the main coronary arteries, aorta ascendens and PT originated in the middle third of the tunica media, passed the external vascular layers, and finally drained into a longitudinal adventitial venous plexus. The latter released small veins which were tributaries of the ventricular coronary veins. There were a few arterio-venous anastomoses in the middle third of the tunica media. The tunica intima and inner third of the tunica media were shown to be avascular.

7 The Anatomy of Veins Draining the Myocardium of Both Atria

Morphologically, ventricular veins have been well studied, but AVs to a lesser degree. In the majority of publications the descriptions of AVs (except the OV) are rather poor and imprecise; moreover, the figures and drawings in the atlases frequently show almost avascular epicardial surfaces of both cardiac atria (Figs. 26, 27).

Some illustrations depict small vascular lumina on the endocardial surface of the right sinus venosus, which are sometimes designated "openings of smallest cardiac veins" (Bargmann 1963; Putz and Pabst 2000).

Questions have also arisen as to whether or not the other very thin, subendocardial cardiac sinuses, tunnels, and channels belong to the SCVS (Rosinia and Low 1986).

Examination of the modern physiological literature also suggests that classification of all small and smallest cardiac veins simply as vv cardiacae minimae may not, anatomically or clinically, be entirely appropriate (Kenner et al. 1984).

According to our findings, the walls of both cardiac atria are drained by three venous systems, the GCVS, the SCVS, and the compound venous system (von Lüdinghausen 1995; von Lüdinghausen et al 2000) (Figs. 26, 27).

1. The GCVS consists of mainly subepicardially (epimurally) distributed veins that open via sinuses into the right and the left atrium. The veins draining the walls of the LA may be divided into the following groups:
   a. Those emptying into the RA (so-called left atrial anteroseptal, posteroseptal, and inferoseptal veins)
   b. Those emptying into the CS (posterior and oblique veins of the LA)
   c. Those emptying into the left coronary vein (left lateral and auricular veins of the LA)
   d. Those emptying into the LA itself (non-coronary proper veins of the LA)
   e. Those emptying into terminal PVs (non-coronary proper veins of the LA)
   f. Those emptying into mediastinal veins (non-coronary extracardiac veins of the LA)
2. There are also numerous vessels of the SCVS which drain the inner layers of the atrial myocardium. Veno-sinusoidal and arterio-sinusoidal vessels connect some intramyocardial venules and arterioles with special intramural "blood pools", which are regarded as very small intramyocardial or intertrabecular sinusoids.
3. The compound venous systems consist of numerous intramural tunnels or spaces. These vessels connect epimurally and intramurally distributed veins.

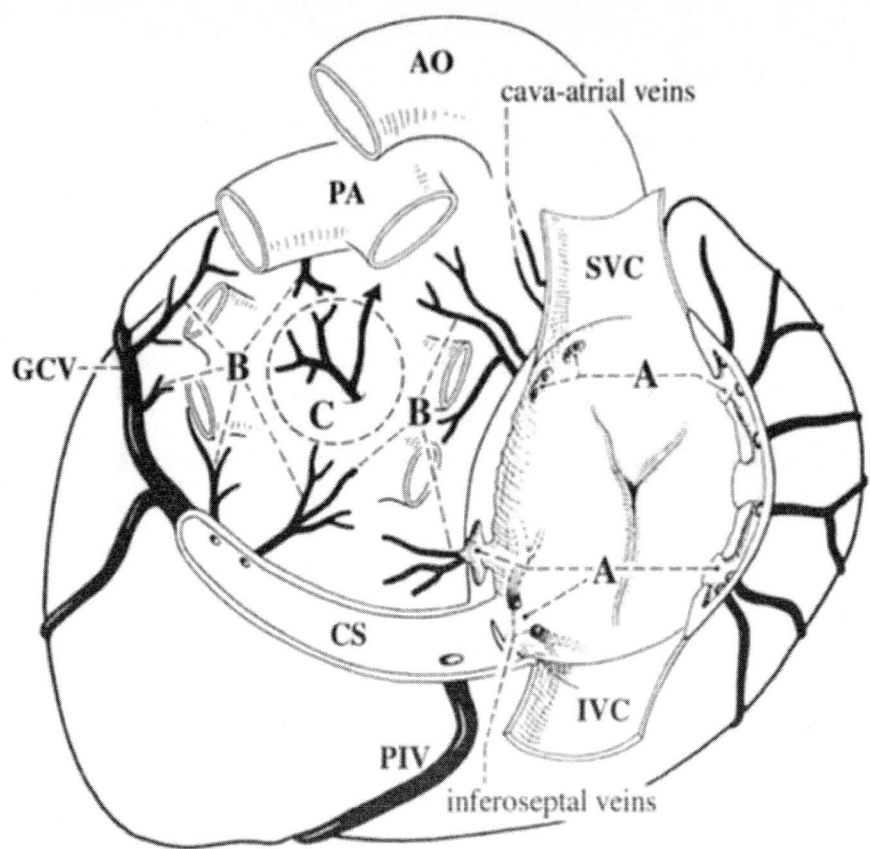

Fig. 26. Schematic drawing of the human heart (dorsolateral aspect) showing the distribution pattern and three modes of openings of the great (major) cardiac veins. *A*: Veins forming intramural (intramyocardial) atrial sinuses and emptying into the RA. *B*: Veins draining the walls of the LA and emptying into the GCV, CS, and RA. *C*: Left atrial veins emptying into the LA and mediastinum (marked by an *arrow*). It appears that there are four ways of left atrial drainage: (1) veins drain into the GCV and CS, (2) veins drain directly into the RA, (3) veins empty directly into the LA, (4) veins pass the bare area of the LA and are connected with mediastinal veins. Cava-atrial and inferoseptal veins are also indicated

7.1
The Veins of the Left Atrium

Three groups of small delicate veins distributed in and on the walls of the LA are frequently found to divide into three groups: (1) posterolateral veins, (2) posterosuperior veins and (3) antero- and posteroseptal veins.

The anatomical distribution pattern and physiological experiments concerning atrial venous drainage reveal that the majority of left atrial veins are tributaries of the GCVS (Gates et al. 1993; von Lüdinghausen et al. 1995; von Lüdinghausen et al. 2000) (Figs. 26, 27, 28).

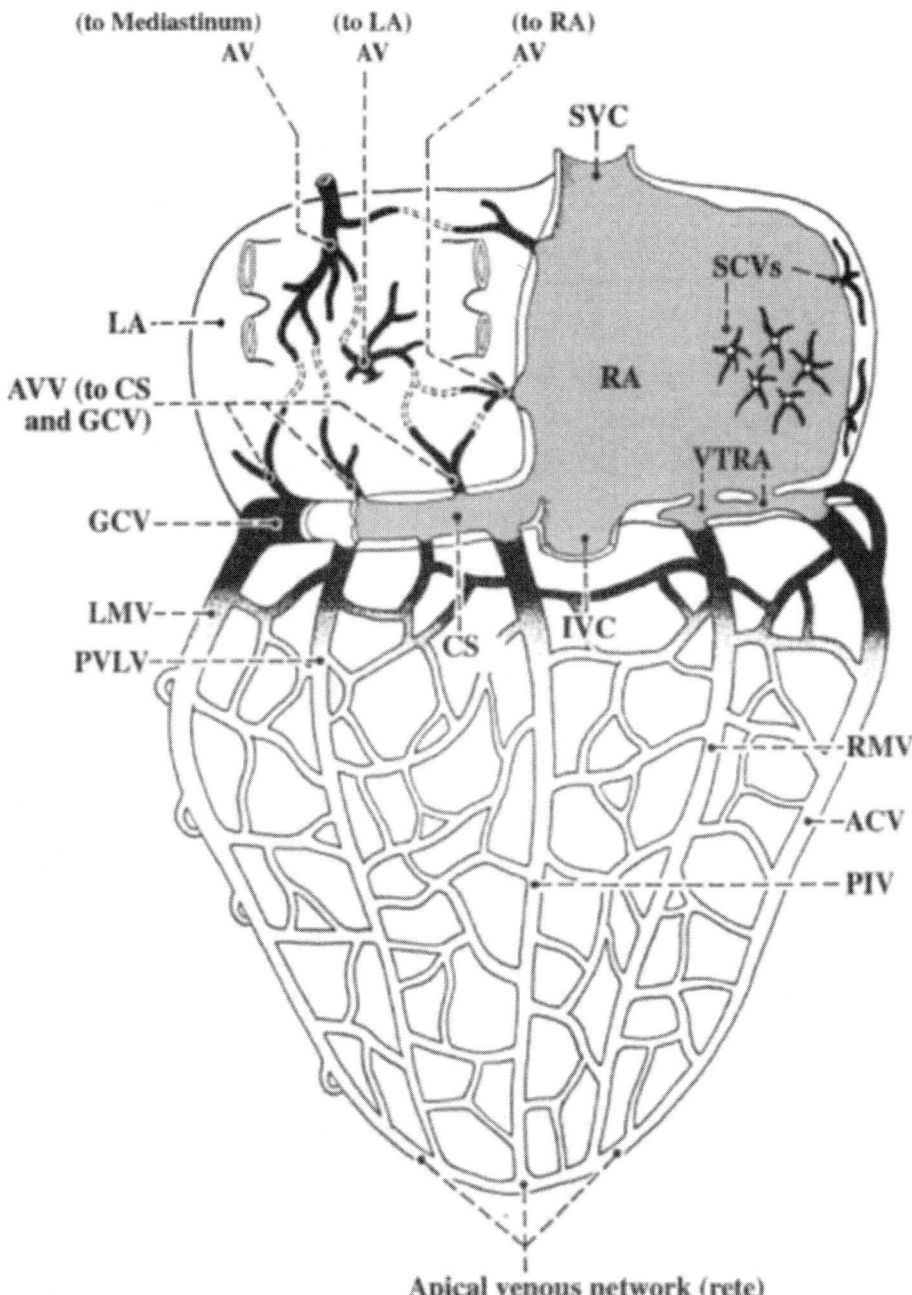

Apical venous network (rete)

Fig. 27. Two-dimensional view of all veins of the greater and smaller cardiac venous system (GCVS and SCVS) illustrating the atrial and ventricular veins, their connections, and atrial openings. The ventricular veins form a venous basket of intercommunicating veins characterized by four or five axially orientated venous stems which have all joined together in the veins or sinuses of the coronary sulcus. In a few cases, an almost complete venous ring may be formed by the CS, the GCV, the SCV, and a long version of the venous tunnel of the right atrium (*VTRA*). The veins of the myocardial walls of the RA and LA exhibit a variable distribution pattern

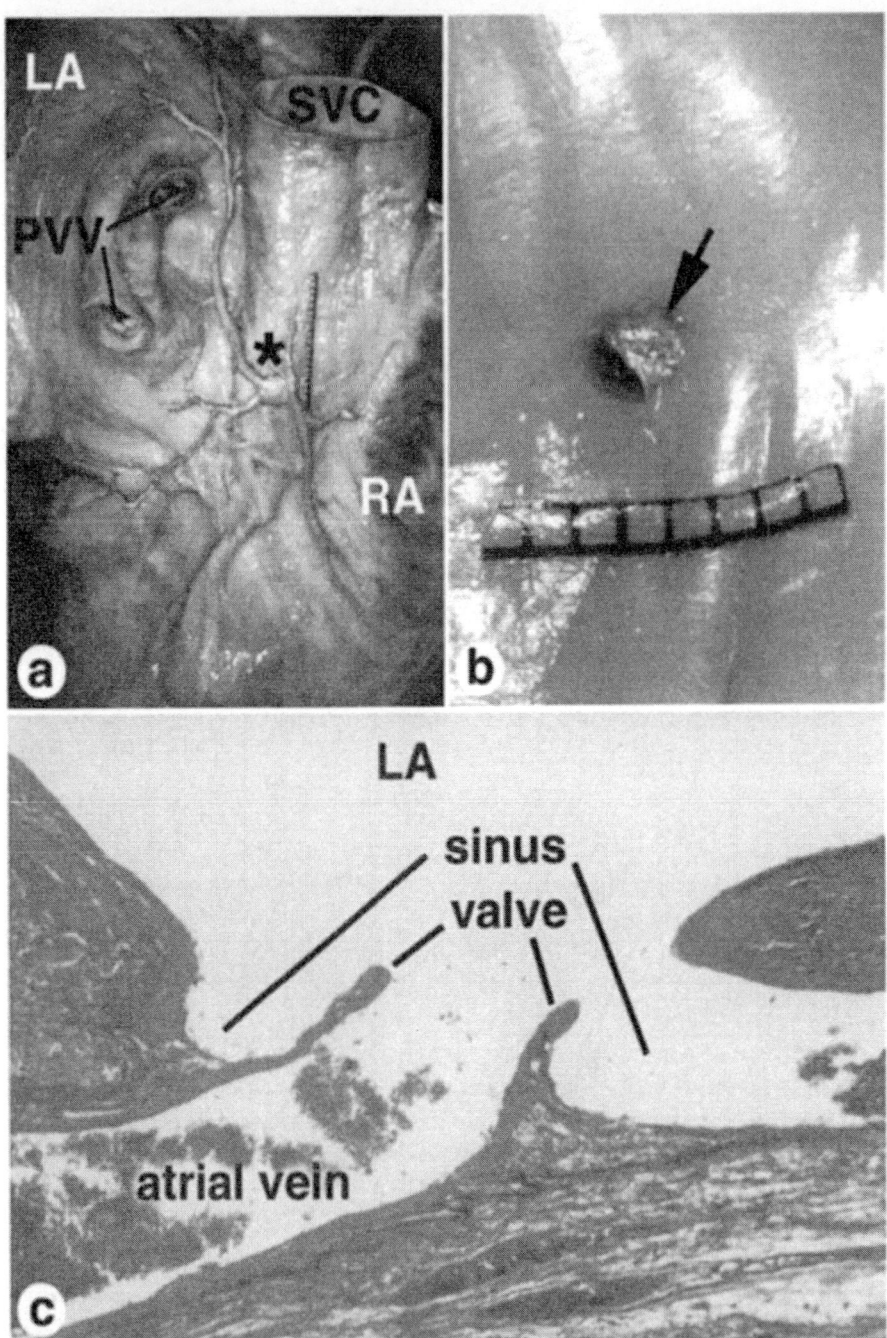

Fig. 28a–c. Left atrial veins and their mode of opening as seen in cadaveric specimens (posterosuperior aspect). a Anteroseptal and posteroseptal veins drain the myocardium in the vicinity of the right PVs and join together to empty into a small intramural sinus (marked by an *asterisk*) which opens into the dorsal wall of the venous sinus of the RA. b Internal posterosuperior wall of the RA showing the unicuspid valve of a left atrial vein in a shallow depression or sinus (marked by an *arrow*). c Histological section of the posterosuperior wall of the LA showing a proper left atrial vein and its ostium which opens into an intramural sinus. The ostium is marked by a bicuspid valve. H&E staining, ×480

7.1.1
Posterolateral Veins of the LA

These veins drain the left posterior and lateral walls of the LA and its auricle. Generally these veins joined the CS, and their pattern of distribution was the same in most of the cases examined:

In 78% of the specimens there was a vein draining the middle and right parts of the posterior wall, and in 99% of the specimens one was draining the left part of the posterior wall of the LA. The latter is commonly known as the OV (see Chap. 6.8 "The Oblique Vein of the Left Atrium"). In their terminal parts, both veins followed intramyocardial courses of 1–4 mm in length (in 12% of the cases) and then opened into the CS. In about 75% of the cases the venous openings had complete unicuspid or bicuspid valves (von Lüdinghausen et al. 1995).

In 5% of the cases the valve observed was not an ostial but an intramural valve, situated 1–5 mm away from the CS, and the terminal part of the vein was noticeably wider. In 20% of the cases no valves were visible.

7.1.2
Posterosuperior Veins of the LA

These veins were present in 74% of the cases and drained the myocardium between the openings of the pulmonary veins, i.e., the posterosuperior wall of the left atrium. There were one, two, or three small veins, which, after a mostly epimural course of 20–30 mm and after collecting some other thin branches, emptied either into the left atrium itself (in 68% of the cases) or more laterally into a terminal part of one of the pulmonary veins (in 5% of the cases).

7.1.3
Anteroseptal and Posteroseptal Veins of the LA

These veins drain the myocardium of the septal region. These empty directly into the RA.

Anteroseptal veins – distributed on the anterior and septal walls of the LA – were found in 99% of our cases. They formed one or two stems, which followed an epimural course to the right, passing the anterior interatrial sulcus to penetrate the myocardium of the RA at the junction of the SVC and the sinus venarum, superior and anterior to the oval fossa. Here, the anteroseptal veins exhibited round, funnel-shaped or slot-like ostia with unicuspid or bicuspid valves (so-called funnel valves according to von Kügelgen 1958). The ostia themselves opened into subendocardial depressions or sinuses with a depth and width of 0.5–1.0 mm, terminating within one or two shallow or deep endocardial depressions, excavations and lacunae of 1.2–3 mm in diameter.

These depressions or intramural sinuses of the RA are also named "sinus septi interatrialis" (Nguyen and Doutriaux 1975). In some cases the sinuses have been found to be marked with perforated translucent laminae.

Posteroseptal veins on the posteroseptal wall of the LA were found in only 34% of the cases examined. One or two veins of that group left the posterior wall of the LA, joined with an interatrial septal branch, crossed the posterior interatrial sulcus and emptied, posterior to the oval fossa, into the RA. One or two subendocardial or intramural sinuses (3–6 mm in length and 1–3 mm in width) were found here, in most cases with cribriform endocardial duplications or laminae, but not by real valves.

These sinuses have been interpreted (by Yater 1929) as remnants of the left valve of the sinus venarum. In 6% of the cases a large posteroseptal vein drained a greater myocardial area and replaced one of the posterior atrial veins.

7.1.4
Ostial Valves of the Anteroseptal and Posteroseptal Veins of the LA

The use of a magnifying glass permitted the identification of bicuspid valves at the ostial openings of these veins in 78% of the cases, and unicuspid valves in 12%. In the remaining 10% of the cases, the venous openings exhibited no valves at all. (Fig. 28 a–c).

7.1.5
Intramural Sinuses of the Atrial Walls

The atrial intramural sinuses were first described by Lannelongue (1867) and are therefore known as the crypts of Lannelongue (Tandler 1913; Tschabitscher 1984). There are a few connections between the sinus septi interatrialis and intramural tunnels or sinus of the myocardial base of the RA (according to Tandler 1913).

7.1.6
Extracardiac Intercommunications

In 32% of the cases, one or two of the posterosuperior veins connected with branches of mediastinal veins (probably bronchial veins), after having passed over the bare area of the LA, also named the porta venosa of the heart (Moore 1985), which is encircled by the epipericardial reflection.

These connections represent an alternative route for venous drainage in cases of venous reperfusion via CS catheterization. The anastomotic connections are found at two locations:
1. On the epipericardial junction of the LA, to connect mediastinal veins and veins of the azygos–hemiazygos system (Ovenfors 1956; von Lüdinghausen et al. 1995).
2. Along the trunks of the great vessels, especially the aorta, the PT, and the SVC, to connect the vascular networks of the vasa vasorum (Baroldi and Scomazzoni 1965). There have been reports of the instance of reverse blood flow from the deep bronchial veins into the LA (Bochdalek 1868; Marchand et al. 1950; Shaner 1961; Horiguchi et al. 1988).

The significance of extracardiac venous anastomoses becomes evident from the following two cases observed in the dissection room:

a. The invasive growth of a central bronchogenic carcinoma, where the pulmonary veins had been occluded and their blood had to be transported from the lungs via enlarged bronchial and atrial veins into the LA and RA

b. Congenital atresia of the atrial ostium of the CS and an absent or only small and narrow persistent left SVC (von Lüdinghausen and Lechleuthner 1988), where the ventricular venous blood had to be drained during the lifetime of the subject via widened and interconnected left and right atrial vessels into the RA

Development

There is a sound developmental and comparative anatomical explanation for the existence of the proper left atrial veins. Grant and Regnier (1926), Halpern (1953), Shaner (1961), Clarke (1965a), and Moore (1988) point out that in rats and in late human ontogenesis, the LA expands and gradually incorporates the single primitive, and later the four definitive, PVs; the terminal parts of the accompanying bronchial veins are also incorporated. However, some of these veins become independent vessels, draining the posterosuperior wall of the LA (Christ 1990).

Peculiarities

In a few cases (5%) there was both an atrial vein and a mediastinal vein with an opening into the LA in the same specimen.

In two cases the superior wall of the LA was drained by a vein consisting of two branches. One emptied into the LA, while the other passed through the cardiac porta venosa and joined a mediastinal vein.

7.2
The Veins of the Right Atrium

In comparison with the walls of the LA, the myocardium of the RA enjoys special venous drainage by (1) small right atrial veins, (2) intramurally distributed venous sinuses and tunnels of the right atrium (VTRA), and (3) inferoseptal venous sinuses (Figs. 26, 27, 28a, 29, 30a–d, 31, 32a–d).

7.2.1
Small Right Atrial Veins

In the subendocardial layers of the openings of both venae cavae into the RA and the subendocardial layers of the walls of the sinus venarum there are a few very small veins and venous tunnels a few millimeters in length and 1 mm in width. These small vessels, found in 73% of our cases (von Lüdinghausen et al. 1995, 2000), terminate in pinhead-sized small excavations. There were translucent unicuspid valves at the internal atrial ostia in about 50% of our cases, although Leonhardt (1987) denies the existence of venous valves.

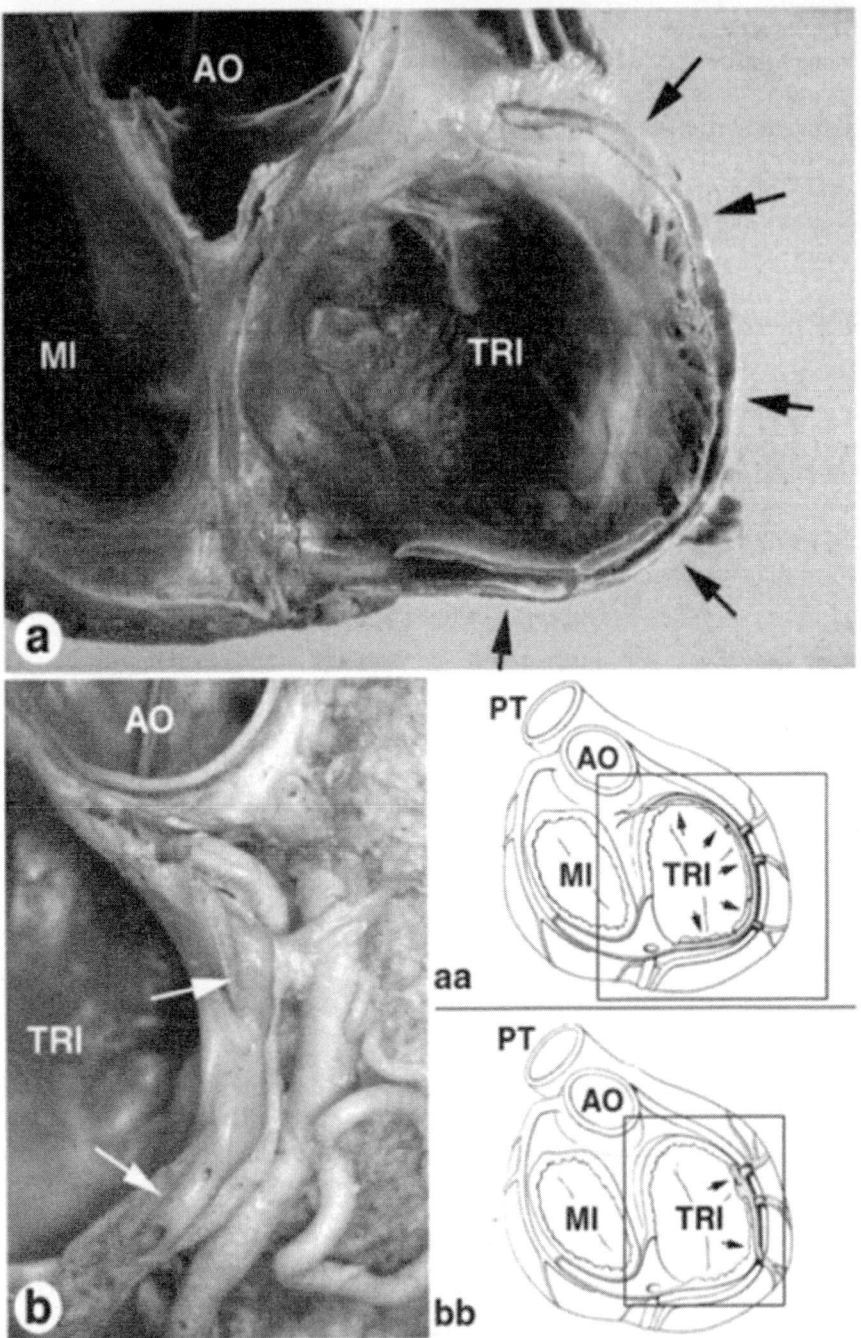

Fig. 29a,b. View of the base of the heart in cadaveric specimens, after removal of nearly all of the atrial walls. Intramural venous tunnels (*VTsRA*) or sinuses of varying lengths can be seen in the anterior and lateral wall of the RA. These frequently occurring sinuses have an almost vertical orientation and run roughly parallel to the fibrous ring of the tricuspid valve. The areas enclosed within rectangles in the schematic drawings correspond to the photographs of the cadaveric specimens. **a** This long VTRA (marked by *arrows*) describes almost two-thirds of a circle, collects most of the ACVs and opens directly into the RA. **b** This short intramural venous sinus (marked by *arrows*) receives three ACVs

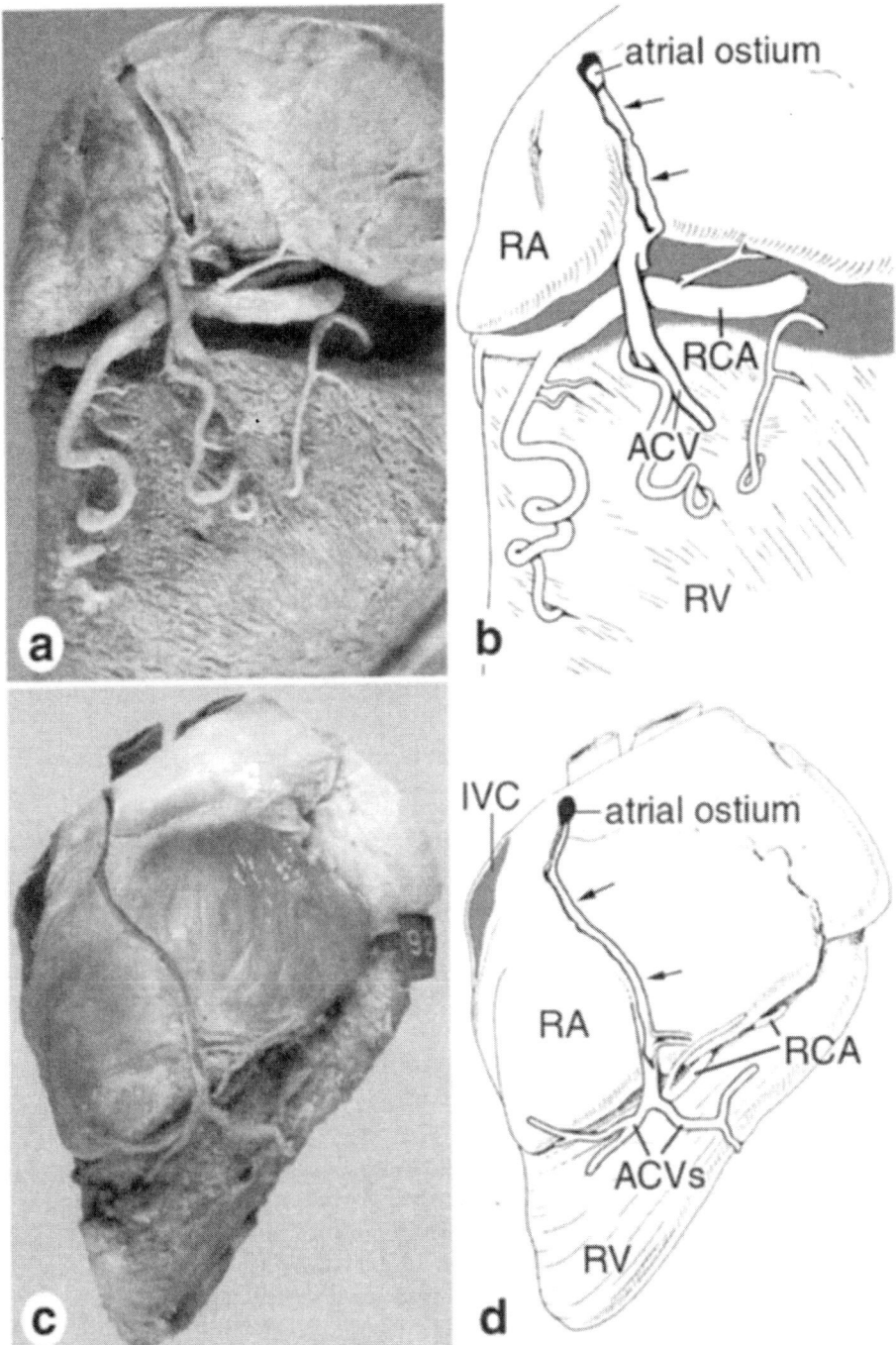

Fig. 30a–d. Transversally orientated intramural venous sinuses of rare occurrence in the anterior and superior walls of the right auricle. Sinuses of this kind constitute the continuation of a common venous stem or trunk which has collected most of the ACVs. The schematic drawings (b and d) correspond to the photographs of the cadaveric specimens. a, b A VTRA of medium length empties into the "roof" of the right auricle. c, d A rather long VTRA empties into the area of the sulcus terminalis at about the midpoint between the ostia of the caval veins

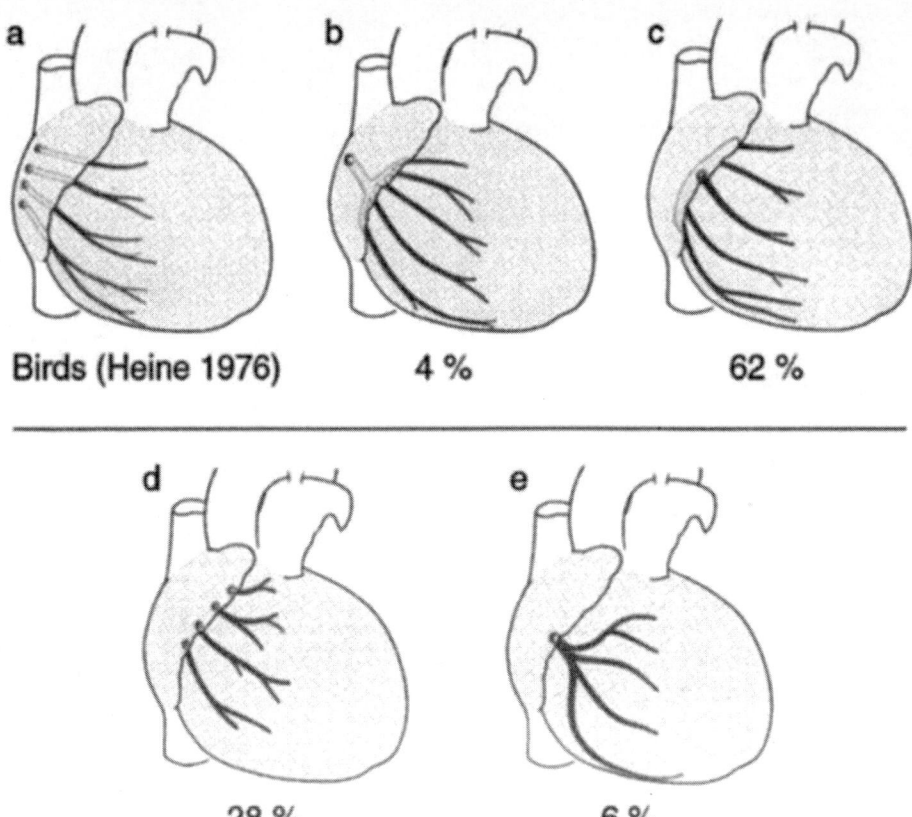

Birds (Heine 1976)   4 %   62 %

28 %   6 %

Fig. 31a–e. Schematic drawing to show the mode and frequency of the distribution pattern of the ACVs in birds (a) and man (b–e). **a** The ACVs reach the RA as single vessels and empty solely between the caval veins (findings according to Heine 1976). **b** The ACVs form a short extramural common stem and intramural sinus which has a transverse orientation and empties solely into the right auricle (frequency 4%). **c** The ACVs empty into an intramural, almost vertically orientated sinus in the anterior wall of the right auricle (frequency 62%). **d** The ACVs open as single vessels directly into the anterior margin of the right auricle (frequency 28%). **e** The ACVs form an extramural common stem which drains directly into the right auricle (frequency 6%)

Lannelongue (1867) and Langer (1880) were the first to demonstrate that small vessels arise from endocardial foramina in the sinus venarum, interconnect the foramina with each other, and also interconnect both the coronary veins and the capillary network in the auricular myocardium. Accordingly, some of these endocardial foramina at the junction of the SVC and the RA are called Lannelongue's endocardial foramina or crypts (Tandler 1926; Tschabitscher 1984) which correspond to the atrial depressions or subendocardial sinuses.

A number of these veins empty into the stems of the left anteroseptal atrial veins.

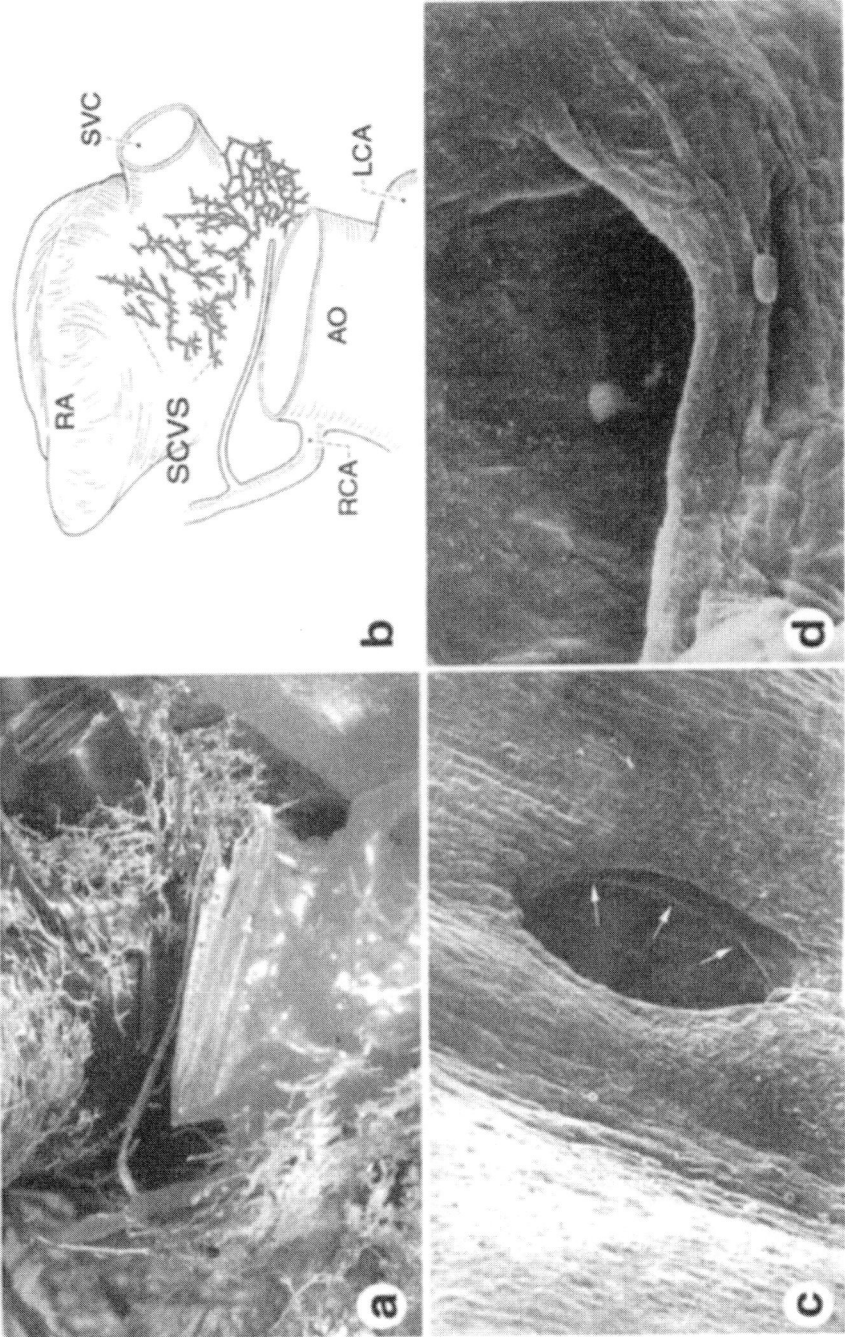

Fig. 32a–d. Distribution pattern and modes of opening of components of the SCVS in the walls of the RA as seen in corrosion cast (a) and in SEM (c and d). a Lateral view of the aortic root, main stems of the coronary arteries and the right auricle. On the left wall of the right auricle, numerous very small vessels can be seen to form a dense network. b Schematic drawing corresponding to a. c The atrial ostium of this smallest cardiac vessel is marked by a small lip-like endothelial fold (*white arrows*) which may act as a valve (of obvious insufficiency). d The atrial ostium of this vessel, which follows an oblique course, is marked by a small (obviously insufficient) unicuspid valve

7.2.2
Venous Drainage of the SA Node

The venous drainage of the area of the SA node is indifferent: a few tiny sinusoids and subendocardial veins are distributed in the region of the sinus node, chiefly at its periphery. Some were seen by Kennel and Titus (1972) to have openings into the smooth walls of the sinus venarum, others emptied into the trabecular meshwork of the adjacent musculi pectinati, and still others opened into the VTRA before they eventually communicated directly with the right atrial cavity. All were thin-walled and lined with a simple flattened endothelium (see next paragraph).

The walls of the right auricle are mostly drained by smallest cardiac vessels, revealed not by dissection, but by casting techniques (Bohning et al. 1933; Unger 1938; Ratajczyk-Pakalska and Kolff 1984; von Lüdinghausen et al. 1995).

The area of the lamina supravalvularis was occasionally drained by small atrioventricular veins which finally join the ACVs.

7.2.3
Venous Drainage of the AV Node and Bundle Area

The region of the AV node and bundle was found to be drained in 55% of our cases by numerous venous sinusoids. There were one or two small venous tunnels up to 3.5 cm long and 1.0 mm wide in the base of the interatrial septum just above the tricuspid valve near to the location of the AV node and bundle (also observed by Truex and Schwarz 1951 and Parsonnet 1953). According to our findings these sinusoids coursed almost parallel to and 2 cm above the tricuspid valve ring and usually opened into the RA near the atrial ostium of the CS directly beneath the ostial valve. On occasion, the ostium of such a sinus was separate from and to the right of the CS ostium. A few atrial openings exhibited threadlike structures, but no definite signs of valves (von Lüdinghausen and Schott 1990).

7.2.4
Venous Tunnel or Sinus of the Right Atrium

The termination of the ACVs (including the right marginal, right conus, and right atrioventricular veins) appears to vary considerably; many of these veins do not open directly into the RA. After crossing over or under the RCA, the ACVs were found to drain into a single subendocardially, intramurally or subepicardially situated venous tunnel or channel (VTRA) which is situated in the anterolateral and/or posterior wall of the right auricle parallel to the right coronary sulcus and 1 or 2 cm above the tricuspid valve ring (Mochizuki 1933; Mierzwa and Kozielec 1975; Nguyen and Doutriaux 1975; Esperenca Pina 1975; von Lüdinghausen et al.1984; von Lüdinghausen and Schott 1990; Ortale and Marquez 1998). The frequency of this pattern in our material was 62%; it was 23% in that of Parsonnet (1953), and 52% in that of Esperanca Pina (1975).

The frequently found VTRA measures 1-12 cm in length and 1-4 mm in diameter. In cases we studied, the longest tunnel ran almost parallel to the right coronary sulcus and formed almost a semicircle. The designation "sinus coronarius atrii dextri" or right venous semicircle (in accordance with Nguyen et al. 1981) has been proposed by von Lüdinghausen and Schott (1990). Such tunnels were previously described by Bochdalek (1868) and their existence confirmed by Langer (1880), but their occurrence seems subsequently to have been forgotten.

7.2.5
The Ostia of the VTRA

According to its length, an intramural venous tunnel or sinus usually bears 1-3 valveless orifices, 1-3 mm in diameter which open into the RA near the right margin between the musculi pectinati; we observed a single ostium in 31%, two ostia in 59%, and three ostia in 9% of our cases. In other cases the opening of an intramural sinus was located just within the ostium of the CS, directly beneath its atrial valve. In a few instances the ostium of such a venous sinus was found to be separate from, and to the right of, the orifice (ostium) of the CS. (Mochizuki 1933; Baroldi and Scomazzoni 1965; McAlpine 1975; Tschabitscher 1984).

7.2.6
Topographical Relationship of the VTRA

In topographical terms, such a venous tunnel, sinus or channel lay just above the supravalvular lamina of the auricle, in a position roughly parallel to the coronary sulcus and the fibrous annulus of the tricuspid valve and at a right angle to the course of the anterior cardiac veins (McAlpine 1975; von Lüdinghausen 1987). In 15% of the cases the VTRA was only partly embedded in the right auricular myocardium; here, about one-third or even one-half of the length was constructed from smooth muscle fibers in a fashion similar to that of a normal venous wall (Mochizuki 1933; von Lüdinghausen et al. 1984).

In view of their topographical relationship, these sinuses belong to the compound type of the cardiac venous system.

Peculiarities

In a few cases the sinuses anastomosed with a SCV, which thereafter emptied into the terminal PIV or directly into the RA.

In 3% of our cases the intramural sinus did not follow a course parallel to the coronary sulcus but ran almost vertically through the atrial myocardium in the direction of the ostium of the SVC.

In three out of seven cases (studied by Parsonnet 1953) where a VTRA was present, there was also a SCV, which argues against these veins being identical.

7.2.7
Explanation for the Existence of the VTRA

Many authors find the existence of a right atrial venous tunnel difficult to explain. Where there is a posterior VTRA, one assumption is that the SCV may have migrated from the posterior coronary sulcus and been integrated into the posterior atrial wall. However, there are a few cases where a VTRA was present and also a SCV (see previous paragraph). Where there is an anterior VTRA, one can assume that the ACVs need – for the same hemodynamic reason as the left ventricular veins need the CS – an intramural spacious collector or blood pool before emptying into the RA.

Alternatively, the fetal form of venous drainage into the RA may have been effected through intramural tunnels or sinuses.

According to our findings, there are five modes of course of the ACVs in the walls of the RA (Fig. 31a–e):
1. In birds, the ACVs form four to five vertically oriented intramural sinuses before opening into the RA (Heine 1976).
   In the human:
2. The ACVs open into one vertically oriented intramural sinus, which in turn opens into the RA (in 3% of our specimens: von Lüdinghausen et al. 1995).
3. The ACVs empty in an intramural sinus parallel to the coronary sulcus; the sinus itself opens by means of two orifices into the RA (in 62% of our specimens).
4. The ACVs collect together into one vein that empties into the RA (in 28% of our specimens.
5. The ACVs come together to form a unique stem which crosses the right coronary sulcus and empties into the RA (in 6% of our specimens).

Thus, in some instances there is evidence of a migration of the terminal parts of the ACVs from intramurally situated sinuses to the surface of the RA, where they become freely developed epimural coursing veins.

Peculiarities

In a few of our cases (5%) there was the conspicuous presence of long VTsRA (5–9 cm in length and 2–4 mm in width) parallel to the right coronary sulcus and just above the tricuspid valve (see also Mochizuki 1933; McAlpine 1975; Navaratnam 1975; Nguyen and Doutriaux 1975; Nguyen et al. 1981; Tschabitscher 1984; Waller and Schlant 1994; Ortale and Marquez 1998; Ortale et al 2001). The shorter of these tunnels took the form of an arc imitating either a quarter or a third of a circle, the longer ones described a semicircular ring in the walls of the right auricle (von Lüdinghausen 1987). In the latter instance, the superior opening was situated near the ostium of the SVC and the inferior opening near the ostium of the IVC. (Fig. 29 a,b).

A few VTsRA replaced the SCV. They drained most of the ACVs and the right marginal vein and emptied either into the RA just above the crux cordis or into the terminal part of the CS (see also Mochizuki 1933). In such cases there was no small vein in the posterior coronary sulcus.

A few VTsRA did not run parallel to the coronary sulcus but at a right angle to it; one specimen exhibited a short tunnel (of 11 mm length), another a medium-length tunnel (31 mm), and a third a long tunnel (37 mm). The tunnels began at the right coronary sulcus and ran straight and almost vertically within the myocardium of the right auricle to terminate, not far from the sulcus terminalis and the ostium of the SVC, in the RA (von Lüdinghausen et al 1995)(Fig. 30 a–d.)

Function

It has been assumed, because of their rather frequent occurrence and interconnected distribution pattern, that the VTsRA participate in the myocardial hydraulic system during systole (Lunkenheimer et al.1984). On the other hand, they may support the suction effect of, and venous reflux into, the atria during diastole (Sun et al. 2002).

8 The Significance of the Coronary Sinus and Cardiac Veins in Cardiology

The venous drainage of the coronary vascular bed consists of CS drainage to the RA and non-coronary sinus drainage to both the right and left sides of the heart. The CS functions as a collecting space for the venous blood from the ventricular veins during ventricular systole. Being strongly fixed to the left atrial myocardium, the CS is emptied during atrial systole (Meerbaum 1984; Tsujioka et al. 1984; Sun et al. 2002).

Aside from its important physiological significance, it should be noted that the CS is currently used as a preferential conduit for diagnostic and therapeutic interventions (Figs. 33, 34).

8.1
The Anatomical Basis for Reperfusion of the CS and Selected Cardiac Veins and Imaging of the Coronary Venous Drainage System Using CT

8.1.1
Purpose of Reperfusion Technique

Following the experiments of Beck (1948), Beck and al. (1948), and Mohl (1984b), the CS seems, from the anatomical point of view, to be the ideal location for the placement of a catheter for the purpose of reperfusion or other cardiological procedures (Hochberg and Austen 1980; Grossmann 1985; Mohl et al. 1992).

These procedures include reperfusion for purposes of coronary artery thrombolysis and retroperfusion for the delivery of cardioplegic solutions and sonicated microbubbles used in echocardiographic determination of myocardial blood flow, as well as the positioning of catheters both for pacing during electro-physiological studies and to deliver energy for the disruption of accessory atrioventricular pathways.

8.1.2
Basis of CS Catheterization

Reperfusion techniques of the CS are based on the general assumption, according to physiological experiments, that 95% of the human ventricular myocardium is drained by the CS and its tributaries.

In canine hearts, CS drainage constitutes about 60% of the coronary blood flow (Scharf et al. 1971). The non-coronary sinus channels of the right heart (including the ACVs) account for about 30% of the total venous drainage. According to Scharf et al. (1971), left heart drainage is small, constituting not more than 10% of the outflow.

On the assumption that this is true, the CS is the perfect location for the placement of a catheter for purposes of reperfusion (Hochberg and Austen 1980; Grossmann 1985) carried out with arterial blood or nutritive solutions (Bretschneider 1980; Meerbaum 1984; Mohl 1984b; Yukihoro and Mohl 2000).

The most common pattern of tributaries of the CS is designated a pentad of large veins (Tandler 1926; Mechanik 1934; Hood 1968). However, recent further examination of a large number of heart specimens has not reconfirmed this relatively simple vascular organization.

8.1.3
Failure and Limitation of CS Catheterization

In practical cardiology, there is a failure of catheterization of the CS and cardiac veins in 10%–20% of cases (Frei and Bussmann 1981; Fabiani et al. 1986; Baim 1988), with local subendocardial and mural hemorrhages, disturbances of the conduction system, and perforation of the atrial wall and/or cardiac tamponade. On the strength of these experiences, it is assumed that the procedure of cannulation of the CS and cardiac veins is quite often limited by anatomical variations, irregularities, anomalies, and malformations. A few of these will be demonstrated, covering a wide spectrum of anatomical peculiarities.

A detailed knowledge of the anatomy and variability of the patterns of the CS and its major tributaries may reduce the number of complications and failures which occur as a result of catheter placement, and thus enhance the effectiveness of coronary venous interventions (Loop et al. 1992).

On the strength of these experiences it is assumed that, quite often, the procedure of cannulation of the CS and cardiac veins is limited by anatomical variations, irregularities, anomalies, and malformations. A few of these, constituting a wide spectrum of variations of the CS itself, will be illustrated in the following paragraphs.

The following findings (own material) are worthy of note and require consideration (Fig. 24). Of cases examined:

1. The existence of a PIV was found in 100%.
2. The existence of an AIV was found in 99%.
3. The existence of a PVLV was found in 95%.
4. The existence of an OV was found in 84%.
5. The existence of an SCV was found in only in 36%.

6. The crossing of the AIV or its branches over the GCV was observed in 45% (there is the danger of compression of the vein in cases with severe coronary atherosclerosis).
7. There were variations in the shape and length of the CS.
8. The ostial valves of the GCV and the CS exhibited many peculiarities.

8.1.4
Computed Tomography

Electrocardiogram-triggered electron-beam CT is used to investigate a wide range of cardiac conditions, especially coronary heart disease (Schaffler et al. 2000). Nowadays it is possible to distinguish between coronary arteries, coronary sinus, and cardiac veins on transverse cross-sectional images. In addition, accurate measurements of these vessels and analysis of the topographical situation are also possible and may prevent misinterpretations. Transverse sections through the diaphragmatic part of the heart permit the visualization of the CS with its atrial ostium, as well as the AIV, the PVLV, the PIV, and occasionally the SCV in their variable courses.

8.1.5
Coronary Venography

The CS is, moreover, a good location and guide for coronary venography and selective venous reperfusion techniques (Schumacher et al. 1995; Sun et al. 2002).

Additionally, many other potential uses of the CS make the acquisition of information regarding this structure more important than ever (Silver and Rowley 1988; Sun et al. 2002).

The variable courses and terminations of the many cardiac veins should be established by contrast studies before any diagnostic interventions or even invasive procedures are undertaken (Beck 1948; McAlpine 1975; Mohl 1984b; Baim 1988).

The presence of a large conus vein is of interest, because the related conus artery or a conus branch are important avenues for collateral development in the presence of occlusive disease. Collaterals are often seen in the venous phase of angiography when the veins are also filled with contrast material. A large conus vein might obscure, and possibly be misinterpreted as, an arterial branch serving a collateral role; it may also act as a source of intersystemic collateral between the coronary and anterior venous systems (McAlpine 1975; Mierzwa and Kozielec 1975).

8.1.6
The Significance of Ostial Valves

Through its myocardial coat, the CS functions as a venous collector; its actions correspond to atrial movements. Therefore, the CS is not only developmentally but also functionally a part of the RA. The purpose of the ostial valve of the CS is only to guide the blood flow to the RA rather than to occlude the atrial ostium, since in the healthy individual there is no danger of congestion and reverse blood flow from the

RA into the CS. For this reason, an efficient ostial valve seems unnecessary. Therefore, some subjects exhibit valveless ostia of the CS or the other great veins without having suffered any disadvantages.

These arguments are also valid in the case of an intramural VTRA, which may collect all or a few of the ACVs, and apply to the ostial valves of the GCV and PIV, which of necessity do not need to be completely occluded.

8.1.7
The Significance of the Smallest Cardiac Vessels

The smallest cardiac vessels and the related subendocardial sinusoids are intensively interconnected with the vessels of the myocardial microcirculation.

The smallest cardiac vessels may be clinically significant in three ways:
1. They may function as a spatial reserve for the hydraulic system of the ventricles during systole (Lunkenheimer et al. 1984) (see next paragraph).
2. They may act as alternative routes of coronary circulation. These routes may reduce or minimize the size of ischemic myocardium; even revival of an area of infarction has been reported (Waller and Schlant 1994).
3. During open-heart surgery (such as valve replacement) they may support in-tramyocardial microcirculation after arterialization of the ischemic myocardium via the CS and coronary veins using arterial blood or nutrient solutions. Thus, the smallest cardiac vessels may play a significant role in the retrograde nourishment of the myocardium; this has been successfully demonstrated both in experiments (Bohning et al. 1933; Schaper and Schaper 1977) and clinically (Mohl 1984b, 2000; Meerbaum 2000).

8.1.8
Concept of the Hydraulic System of the Intramural
and Subendocardial Sinuses in the Cardiac Walls
and in the Heart Chambers

The terminal venous sinuses and the ostial valves of the tributaries of the GCVS are thought to facilitate the return of cardiac venous blood from the myocardium to the right atrial cavity.

In the adult, venous drainage of the ventricular walls takes place during systolic contraction, whereby the capillary blood is pushed either centrifugally into the subepicardially distributed large veins, or centripetally into the subendocardially distributed vessels of the SCVS.

All venous sinuses, the many smallest cardiac veins, and also the small subendo-cardial sinusoids in the subendocardial layers may (following Lunkenheimer et al. 1984) represent a hydraulic system and thus favor the actions of the ventricles during systole. The CS and the many rather large excavations, intramural sinuses, and tunnels in the right atrial walls enhance the diastolic suction effect within the atria (von Lüdinghausen et al. 2000).

Hammond and Austen (1967) discovered that 49% of the total coronary artery flow is drained by the CS and 24% by the ACVs which enter the RA. Thus, the GCVS effects

73% of venous drainage (Hochberg and Austen 1980). These values constitute the basis for the procedure of reperfusion of the CS and its tributaries.

Catheterization of the CS bears the risk of insufficiency or failure when structural peculiarities in the venous outflow hamper the catheter tip and the perfusate itself does not find the ventricular ischemic area.

The unpredictable distribution patterns of the predominantly non-coronary and extracardiac right and left atrial veins make reperfusion techniques of the atrial myocardium (most particularly the sinuatrial node and atrio-ventricular node areas) unsuccessful where the complete prevention of ischemia is concerned (Boekstegers et al. 1994). A number of anatomical peculiarities are worthy of mention (Arom and Emery 1992).

8.2
Anatomical Peculiarities Supporting Venous Reperfusion via the CS

Due to the existence of the many (subepicardial and extracardiac) valveless anastomoses of the major cardiac veins, the boundaries of the drainage areas are not strictly defined but are seen to "overlap." In particular, the anastomoses between the ACVs and the tributaries of the CS are numerous and extensive; thus, venous drainage of the myocardium in cases treated by CS catheterization is guaranteed.

Although all the blood in the CS appears to originate essentially from the left coronary artery, not all the left coronary inflow leaves by this channel. Measurements made by Gregg and Shipley (1947) revealed that "only" 64%–83% of the blood from the left coronary artery drained through the CS (determined during temporary occlusion of the right coronary artery); the remainder was drained by vessels of the SCVS.

8.3
Anatomical Hindrances to Catheterization of the CS and of Cardiac Veins

In 22% of the cases we investigated, the CS collected most of the ventricular veins. In these cases it suggested itself as an ideal location for any reperfusion procedure. However, the catheters placed permanently or temporarily in the CS must be fixed by an inflated catheter balloon. This means that for anatomical reasons, in the majority of cases the SCV, the PIV and the PVLV, and the related myocardium - mainly of the right ventricle - cannot be perfused (von Lüdinghausen and Ohmachi 2001). A possible solution to this dilemma could be the selective catheterization of any cardiac vein in question (von Lüdinghausen 1987; Waller and Schlant 1994) (Figs. 33, 34).

Where the catheterization of the RA, the CS, and the cardiac veins and the subsequent venous reperfusion are concerned, the possible existence of numerous anatomical hindrances or peculiarities must be taken into consideration.

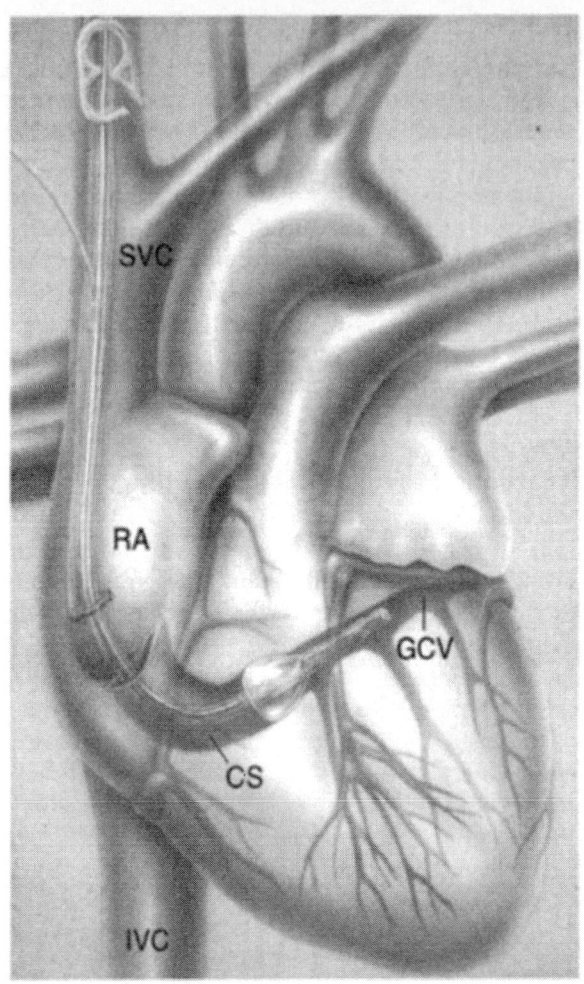

Fig. 33. Anterior aspect of a heart with the cardiac chambers (depicted as transparent) showing the catheterization of the CS via the SVC and RA and placement of a Buckberg Coronary Sinus Cardioplegia Cannula (Research Medical Inc., Research Industries Corporation, 1847 West 2300 South, Salt Lake City, Utah 84119, USA)

8.3.1
The Ostial Valve of the IVC

An unusual net-like ostial valve of the IVC was first observed by Chiari (1897) and subsequently designated as "Chiari's network"; it occurred in 6% of the cases we examined. Yater (1936) found it in 2%–3% of his cases. In topographical terms, between three and twelve thread-like fibrous cords run from the edge of the ostial valve of the CS to the upper extremity of the crista terminalis (Wright et al. 1948; Hickie 1956; Goebel and Gander 1978). Such threads in the ostium of the IVC (as in the ostial valve of the CS) are incomplete remnants of the right valve or septum of the sinus venosus. Prominent ostial valves of the IVC and CS may divide the RA into two parts (Trento et al. 1988) (Fig. 35).

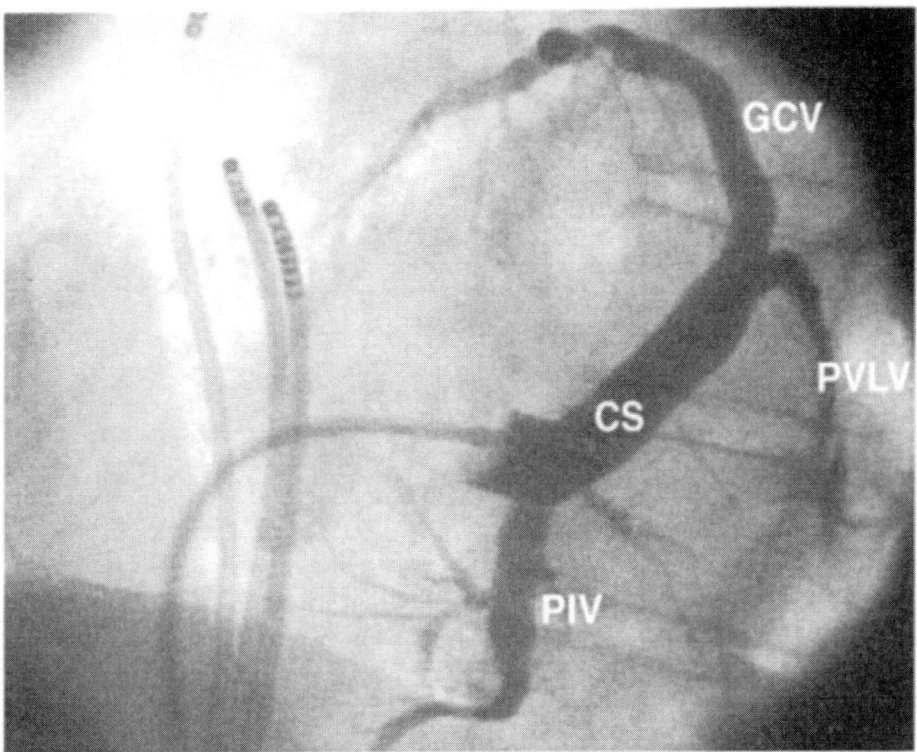

Fig. 34. Angiographically visualized CS and its major tributaries (reprinted with kind permission from Sun et al. 2002)

8.3.2
Persistent Left SVC

The existence of a persistent left SVC emptying into the CS will render any retrograde perfusion of the latter a useless procedure. In such a case, selective catheterization of cardiac veins is indicated.

8.3.3
Aneurysm of the RA, Aneurysm of the CS

In 6% of our cases there was an aneurysm-like excavation or bag, which is known as the posterior auricular appendix or subeustachian sinus of Keith, at the inferior wall of the right atrium (McAlpine 1975; Tschabitscher 1984; Sun et al. 2002). This pocket-like excavation was situated between the orifice of IVC and inferior part of the sulcus terminalis. The largest pseudoaneurysm was 2 cm in width and 2 cm in depth and hung over the crux cordis and its vessels. Characteristically, it had an extremely thin wall (see also Gorlin 1968; Frei and Bussmann 1981).

According to Sun et al. (2002), a pseudoaneurysm of the posterior auricular appendix was also seen in 30% of their cases which exhibited accessory conduction path-

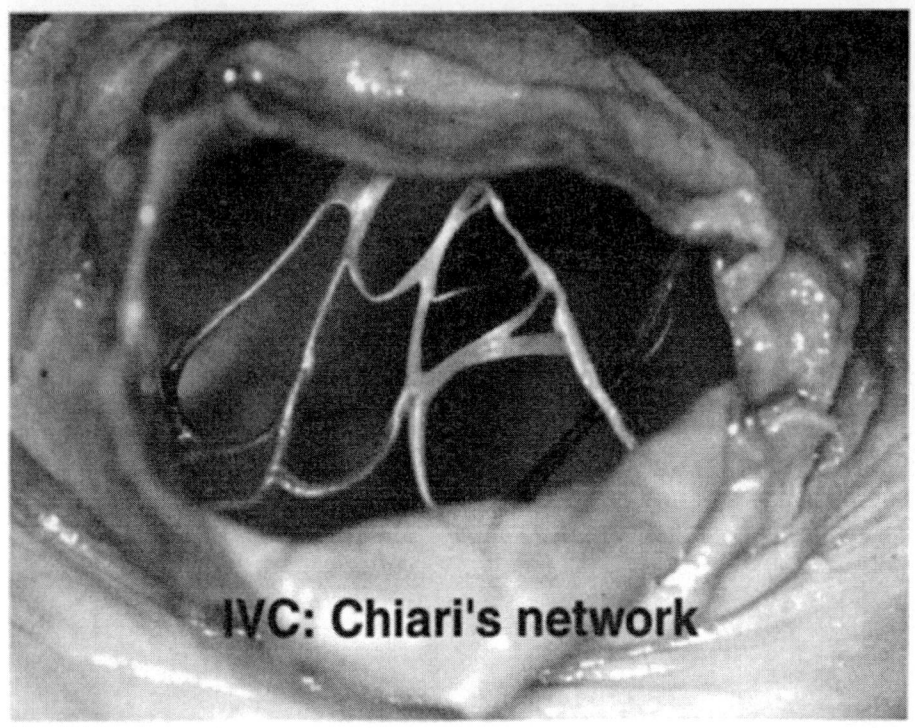

IVC: Chiari's network

Fig. 35. Cross-section of the terminal IVC (seen from inferior): the cribriform network of numerous interconnected endocardial threads (the so-called Chiari's network) is a remnant of the ostial valve of the IVC

ways as in WPW syndrome. It has been suggested that the reason for this coincidence is attributable to a special function of the myocardial coat of the CS.

In rare cases, an aneurysm-like dilation of the CS may be found, mimicking a pericardial tumor (Wenger and Zandanell 1969) (see also Chap. 4.7).

(Pseudo)aneurysms of the RA and CS may increase the risk of perforation during right atrial catheterization.

8.3.4
Rigid Ostial Valves of the CS and GCV

In single cases there may be a rigid membranous or fenestrated ostial valve of the CS preventing any catheterization of the CS.

A complete uni- or bicuspid terminal valve of the GCV or an ostial valve of a large collecting vein may also present a hindrance to the catheter tip during the selective catheterization of cardiac veins. In rare instances, a complete bicuspid valve of the GCV may exhibit a broad, firm commissural mound between the free margins of the cusps. However, in most cases the terminal bicuspid valves are incomplete and, therefore, obviously insufficient (Figs. 8a–c, 10a–d).

8.3.5
Congenital Occlusion of the Atrial Ostium
of the CS

A complete congenital occlusion of the atrial ostium of the CS – combined with a persistent left superior vena cava – may be found incidentally in a cadaveric heart specimen. Such a membranous obstruction of the CS ostium will block any catheterization and perfusion of cardiac veins (von Lüdinghausen and Lechleuthner 1988) (Fig. 10a,b).

8.3.6
Openings of the PIV and PVLV Near to the Atrial Ostium
of the CS

Usually the openings of the PIV and PVLV are situated near to the atrial ostium of the CS. This means that for anatomical reasons, in a case of catheterization of the CS, these two veins cannot be perfused.

8.3.7
The ACVs and the RMV Empty Directly
into the RA

In cases where the ACVs and the RMV empty directly into the RA, the retrograde perfusion of the anterior and posterior wall of the right ventricle by CS catheterization cannot be carried out (Fig. 24).

8.3.8
Opening of the PIV Directly into the RA

Very rarely, the PIV opens directly into the RA. In such a finding, there is a special drainage opening between the two layers of the ostial valve of the CS. The vessel cannot be reached by the perfusate (Figs. 8a, 14).

8.3.9
The Anterior Interventricular Artery Crosses
over the GCV

In 31% of the cases examined, the possibly atherosclerotic anterior interventricular branch crosses over the GCV or its branches and may compress the vein where it courses through the junction of the anterior interventricular sulcus and left part of the coronary sulcus (Fig. 15a,b).

8.3.10
Intramyocardial Course of the AIV

In rare cases there is a short intramyocardial course of the AIV; such a course does not correspond with an intramural course of the anterior interventricular artery. Thus, the intramural part of the vein might be compressed, or even interrupted, during systole (Fig. 17a,b).

8.3.11
Uni- or Bicuspid Valves of the Anterior
and Posterior Septal Veins

Well-developed uni- or bicuspid ostial valves of the anterior and posterior septal veins may prevent adequate retroperfusion of the interventricular septal myocardium (von Lüdinghausen 1987) (Fig. 23a,b).

8.3.12
Ectopic Origin and Aberrant Course of the AIV

An ectopic origin and aberrant course of the AIV with direct opening into the RA will cause the failure of selective venous angiography of the AIV and catheterization and venous reperfusion of the myocardium of the anterior wall of the LV and of the IV septum (Fig. 18a,b).

9 The Cardiac Venous System Seen Three-Dimensionally: An Arrangement of Veins Which Favors Reperfusion Efficacy

All specimens exhibit large, axially orientated venous stems which arise from the apical venous network and course in the IV sulci and at the right and left margins to the coronary sulcus. Here these stems continue into coronary veins or sinuses. These main routes of cardiac venous drainage are interconnected by numerous collateral channels. Parsonnet (1953) described two constant venous anastomotic rings surrounding the right and left ventricles. Additionally, in 34% of our cases an incomplete venous ring was formed in the waist of the heart. This ring consisted of the GCV, the CS, the SCV, and the VTRA.

Seen three-dimensionally, a basket-like or spheroid venous network of variable size may be designated (see Chap. 6.20 "Venous Anastomoses").

All these large and small epicardial veins function together as storage spaces which collect the venous blood on its way from the capillary network to the right atrium (Lechleuthner and von Lüdinghausen 1986). Given the latter, the arrangement and communication of the cardiac veins might be thought to favor the epimural distribution of any perfusate and its drainage. The image of a venous basket – whose parts surround both the ventricles and atria – suggests that all myocardial territories enjoy the same venous drainage capability. However, venous drainage varies individually between the left and right ventricles and left and right atria to a great degree. This should be taken into account when coronary venography (Gensini et al. 1965) and/or reperfusion methods are discussed (Fig. 27).

9.1 The Efficiency of Ostial Valves

Ostial valves of the CS and those in the larger veins are usually of uni- or bicuspid venous type; in most hearts the valves appear insufficient (von Lüdinghausen 1987).

However, there does not seem to be any necessity for efficient venous valves. The more important driving force behind the venous outflow – beside the "vis a tergo" of the bloodstream – is the continual massage of the subepicardially distributed veins through the elasticity of the fiber-bundles in the epicardium and pericardium (Kenner et al. 1984).

Anderhuber (1984) pointed out that valves are found in the longer sections of a cardiac vein and its ramifications. Whether there is adequate development of complete valves in the cardiac veins during the embryonic stage that later (after birth) become insufficient, or whether valve insufficiency has already developed by the time of birth, remains unknown.

The (ostial) terminal valve of the GCV seems in every case to be congenitally insufficient because, when it is a bicuspid valve, the fixation points (commissure) of the cusps are inserted at a distance of 1 or 2 mm from each other; when it is a unicuspid valve, the cusp is able to fill only half of the diameter of the vein (von Lüdinghausen 1987; von Lüdinghausen et al. 2000).

9.2
Prospect

There are three cardiac venous systems: the GCVS, the SCVS, and the compound system of cardiac vessels. Each system contributes to the venous drainage of the myocardium. However, where a natural reverse blood flow during the diastolic phase of heart action is concerned, each system may also participate in the retrograde supply and nutrition of the interior layers of the atrial and ventricular myocardium. The possible nutrition of the internal layers of the myocardium, where there is ramification of the right and left bundle branches through the smallest cardiac vessels and connected intramural veins, may contribute to the recovery of the heart from conduction system irregularities (from fibrillation or simple arrest without fibrillation). The nutrition of myocardium through smallest cardiac vessels affords a reasonable explanation why, for months or even years, the cardiac tissues have, in many cases, survived the obstruction of terminal arteries long believed to be their sole supply. Consequently, an exact consideration of the three systems constitutes the basis for invasive and non-invasive diagnostics and treatment of numerous heart diseases.

In particular, the widespread clinical practice of catheterization of the CS and its tributaries (with the use of retrograde coronary venography and of retrograde delivery of cardioplegic solutions during heart surgery) has led to a decrease in mortality rates and has reduced the costs of cardiac operations; it has, however, led to an increase in the total number of instances of complications. The latter are often due to anatomical peculiarities and anomalies of the CS and cardiac veins that have been described here.

10 Summary

New cardiological techniques such as coronary sinus catheterization and selective catheterization of the cardiac veins permit the opening of new experimental and clinical fields, for instance in venous angiography and the reverse nourishment of myocardium which is endangered by ischemia, and also in the electrophysiological study of the components of the conduction system. New approaches in heart surgery, such as the removal of accessory pathways of the conduction system (as in WPW syndrome), necessitate the realization of the topographical relationships of the vessels in the various sections of the coronary sulci in a different way.

The objective of this work is, therefore, to present comprehensive and almost new macro- and microanatomical data about the venous drainage of the myocardium via the coronary sinus and its related and unrelated (non-coronary) cardiac veins. Examination of meticulously dissected heart specimens (of individuals who had achieved old or extreme old age at the time of their death in Germany; $n=250$) as well as corrosion casts of adult cardiac vessels (of individuals of all ages, $n=25$) formed the basis for the exact description and documentation of the occurrence, frequency, origin, and courses of both the normal and anomalously developed human coronary sinus and cardiac veins. A wide range of morphological and experimental references was consulted in order to enable thorough discussion of the anatomical findings in the light of modern cardiological diagnostics and treatment.

The anatomical and clinical nomenclature is presented and there is a brief comment on modern diagnostic techniques and their applications where the cardiac veins are concerned. The two principal and one compound cardiac venous system are defined and discussed with reference to the existence of both the normal and anomalous coronary sinus and cardiac veins.

1. The greater (major) cardiac venous system
2. The smaller (minor) cardiac venous system
3. The compound cardiac venous system.

The microanatomy of the various proper cardiac veins is not very well explained and illustrated in old or new literature; therefore, special attention is paid in the present study to the detailed microanatomy of the cardiac venous drainage.

This includes the topography and structural and surface anatomy of the coronary sinus (position, length and shape, diameters, area of cross-section, circumference and volume, curvature, elevation, ostial angle, enlargement, duplication, absence), and the exact external and internal morphological landmarks of the coronary sinus with reference to its myocardial cover, isolated myocardial belts, and "free" myocardial cords which connect the atrial and ventricular myocardium, and the atrial ostium of the coronary sinus.

It is established that the frequency, distribution pattern, courses and mode of opening of the major ventricular and atrial cardiac veins and the occurrence, morphology, and efficiency of the ostial valves of the coronary sinus and its tributaries all influence the success of any selective catheter implantation and venous reperfusion technique to a great degree.

There are many peculiarities of the cardiac veins which are worthy of consideration, for instance intramyocardial and aberrant courses of the anterior interventricular vein, the oblique vein of the left atrium, the posterior interventricular vein, the small cardiac vein, the posterior vein of the left ventricle, the left and right marginal veins, and the anterior cardiac veins. Various forms and courses of the intramural venous tunnel, sinus or channel of the right atrium were found and illustrated, and discussed in terms of developmental and comparative anatomy.

This review incorporates a great variety of clinically significant, new morphological findings with regard to the coronary sinus and the cardiac venous system. The many anatomical peculiarities and hindrances to the catheterization of the coronary sinus and the reperfusion of (even selected) cardiac veins are documented and evaluated: the various problems which may arise in venous reperfusion due to the presence of anatomical anomalies of the coronary sinus, cardiac veins, and ostial valves (of greater or lesser efficiency) are addressed.

The presentation narrows a gap in the rather incomplete knowledge of the venous drainage of the human myocardium.

References

Abernethy J (1798) Observations on the Foramina Thebesii of the heart. Philos. Transactions Royal Soc London 88: 103-109

Aho A (1950) On the venous network of the human heart. Ann Med Exper Biol Fenniae 28: Suppl. I

Anderhuber F (1984) Venenklappen in den großen Wurzelstämmen der Vena cava superior. Acta Anat 119: 184-192

Anderson BG, Anderson WD (1981) Myocardial microvasculature studied by microcorrosion casts. Biomed Research 2 (Suppl): 209-217

Anderson RH, Becker AE (1982) Anatomie des Herzens. Thieme, Stuttgart, pp 129-131

Ansari A (2001) Anatomy and clinical significance of ventricular Thebesian veins. Clin Anat 14: 102-110

Arom KV, Emery RW (1992) Retrograde cardioplegia: detail for coronary sinus cannulation technique. Ann Thorac Surg 53: 714-715

Baim DS (1988) Percutaneous placement of coronary sinus catheters. 3rd International Symposium on myocardial protection via the coronary sinus. June 23-24 Cambridge MA, USA (Abstract)

Bankl H (1977) Congenital malformations of the heart and great vessels. Urban & Schwarzenberg, Baltimore, Munich, pp 198-220

Bargmann W (1963) Blutgefässe des Herzens. In: Bargmann W, Doerr W (eds) Das Herz des Menschen, Bd 1. Thieme, Stuttgart, pp 137-146

Baroldi G, Scomazzoni G (1965) Coronary circulation in the normal and the pathologic heart. Armed Forces Institute of Pathology, Office of the Surgeon General, Department of the Army, Washington D.C., pp 5-73

Beck CS (1948) Revascularisation of the heart. Ann Surg 128: 854-864

Beck CS, Leighninger DS (1954) Operations for coronary artery disease. JAMA 156: 1226-1233

Beck CS, Stanton E, Batiuchok W, Leiter E (1948) Revascularisation of the heart by a graft of systemic artery into the coronary sinus. JAMA 137: 436-442

Becker AE, Anderson RH, Durrer D, Wellens HJJ (1978) The anatomical substrates of Wolff-Parkinson-White syndrome. Circulation 57: 870-879

Berg R (1963) Über das Auftreten von Myokardbrücken über den Koronargefäßen beim Schwein. Anat Anz 112: 25-31

Bergman RA, Thompson SA, Saadeh FA (1988) Absence of the coronary sinus. Anat Anz 166: 9-12

Bochdalek Jun (1868) Zur Anatomie des menschlichen Herzens. Arch Anat Physiol 302-325

Boekstegers P, Peter W, von Degenfeld G, Nienaber CA, Abend M, Rehders TC, Habazettl H, Kapsner T, von Lüdinghausen M, Werdan K (1994) Preservation of regional myocardial function and myocardial oxygen tension during acute ischemia in pigs: comparison of selective synchronized suction and retroinfusion of coronary veins to synchronized coronary venous retroperfusion. J Amer Coll Cardiol (JACC) 23: 459-469

Bohning A, Jochim K, Katz LN (1933) The Thebesian vessels as a source of nourishment for the myocardium. Amer J Physiol 106: 183-200

Bretschneider HJ (1980) Myocardial protection. Thorac Cardiovasc Surgeon 28: 295-302

Chiari H (1897) Über Netzbildungen im rechten Vorhofe des Herzens. Beitr Pathol Anat Allg Path 22: 1-10

Christ B (1990) Grundlagen der embryonalen Gefäßbildung. In: Hinrichsen (ed) Human embryology, Springer Berlin, Heidelberg, New York, pp 247-248

Clarke JA (1965a) An X-ray microscopic study of the pattern and distribution of capillary beds in the atria of the human heart. Z Anat Entw Gesch 124: 471–477

Clarke, JA (1965b) An x-ray microscopic study of the vasa vasorum of the normal human pulmonary trunk. Acta Anat 61: 6–14

Cox JL, Ferguson Jr TB (1989) Surgery for the Wolff-Parkinson-White Syndrome: the endocardial approach. Sem Thoracic Cardiovasc Surg 1: 34–46

Dusek J, Ostadal B, Duskova M (1975) Postnatal persistence of spongy myocardium with embryonic blood supply. Arch Pathol 99: 312–317

Edwards JE (1960) Anomalies of the coronary sinus. In: Gould SE (ed) Pathology of the heart, 2nd edn, Thomas Springfield, Ill., pp 431–437

Esperance Pina JA, Dos Santos Ferreira (1974) Microangiographic aspects of the Thebesian veins. Acta Anat 88: 156–160

Esperanca Pina JA (1975) Morphological study on the human anterior cardiac veins, venae cordis anteriores. Acta Anat 92: 145–159

Esperanca Pina JA, Trindade AM (1977) Étude microangiographique des vaisseaux artério-luminaux. Acta Anat 98: 334–339

Feneis H, Dauber W (1998) Anatomisches Bildwörterbuch, 8th edn. Thieme, Stuttgart, pp 186–187

Fleischhauer K (ed) (1985) Das Herz. In: Benninghoff Makroskopische und mikroskopische Anatomie des Menschen, Bd 2, Kreislauf und Eingeweide, 13/14th edn, Urban & Schwarzenberg München, pp 44–79

Foale RA, Baron DW, Rickards AF (1979) Isolated congenital absence of the coronary sinus. Brit Heart J 42: 355–358

Frank CG, Maloney JV (1968) Surgical significance of congenital anomalies of the coronary sinus. J Cardiovasc Surg 9: 420–427

Friedell A (1966) Utilisation of Thebesian blood flow in treatment of coronary heart disease. Minnisota Medicine 49: 1721–1722

Frei U, Bussmann WD (1981) Die Herzbeuteltamponade, eine meist tödliche Komplikation zentraler Venenkatheter. Dtsch Med Wschr 106: 835–837

Frick H (1987) Brusteingeweide. In: Frick H, Leonhardt H, Starck D (eds) Spezielle Anatomie II, 3rd edn. Thieme Stuttgart, pp 25–45

Gates RN, Laks H, Drinkwater DC, Pearl JM, Zaragoza AM, Lewis W, Sorensen TJ, Kaczer EM, Chang PA (1993) Gross and microvascular distribution of retrograde cardioplegia in explanted human hearts. Ann Thorac Surgery 56: 410–416

Gensini GG, di Giorgi S, Coskun O, Palacio A, Kelly AE (1965) Anatomy of the coronary circulation in living man. Circulation 31: 778–784

Gerlis LM, Gibb JL, Williams GJ, Thomas GDH (1984) Coronary sinus orifice atresia and persistent left superior vena cava. Br Heart J 52: 648–653

Giebel J, Fanghänel J, Hauser S, Paul I (2000) A case of a persistent left vena cava superior with atresia of the right atrial ostium. Ann Anat 182: 191–194

Goebel N, Gander MP (1978) Septierung des rechten Vorhofs durch eine große Valvula Eustachii. Fortschr Röntgenstr 129: 389–390

Goerttler K (1963) Entwicklungsgeschichte des Herzens. In: Bargmann W, Doerr W (eds) Das Herz des Menschen, Bd 1, Thieme, Stuttgart, pp 21–83

Gorlin R (1968) Perforations and other cardiac complications. Circulation 37/38 (Suppl): 36–38

Gould SE (1953) Pathology of the heart. CC Thomas, Springfield Ill, pp 549–555

Grant RT (1926) Development of the cardiac coronary vessels in the rabbit. Heart 13: 261–271

Grant RT, Regnier M (1926) The comparative anatomy of the cardiac coronary vessels. Heart 13: 285–317

Grant RT, Viko LE (1929) Observations on the anatomy of the Thebesian vessels of the heart. Heart 15: 103–129

Gregg DE, Dewald D (1938) Immediate effects of coronary sinus ligation on dynamics of coronary circulation. Proc Soc Exper Biol Med 39: 202–204

Gregg DE, Shipley RE (1947) Studies of the venous drainage of the heart. Amer J Physiol 151: 13–25

Gregg DE, Fisher LC (1963) Blood supply of the heart. In: Field J, Magoun HW (eds) Handbook of Physiology, Amer Physiol Soc, Washington D.C., pp 1517–1584

Grossmann W (1985) Cardiac catheterisation and angiography, 3rd edn, Lea & Febiger, Philadelphia, pp 4-29

Gschwend T (1931) Das Herz des Wildschweins. Anat Anz 72: 49-89

Halpern MH (1953) Extracoronary cardiac veins in the rat. Amer J Anat 92: 307-328

Hammond GL, Austen WG (1967) Drainage patterns of coronary arterial flow as determined from the isolated heart. Amer J Physiol 212: 1435-1440

Heine H (1976) Stammes- und Entwicklungsgeschichte des Herzens lungenatmender Wirbeltiere. Abh Senckenberg Naturforsch Ges 535: 1-152

Heintzberger CFM (1984) The vascularisation pattern in the ventricular wall in different species during development. In: Mohl W, Wolner E, Glogar D (eds) The coronary sinus. Steinkopff Darmstadt, Springer New York, pp 47-52

Hellerstein HK, Orbison JL (1951) Anatomic variations of the orifice of the human coronary sinus. Circulation 3: 514-523

Hickie JB (1956) The valve of the inferior vena cava. Brit Heart J 18: 320-326

Hochberg MS, Austen WG (1980) Selective retrograde coronary venous perfusion. Ann Thorac Surg 29: 578-588

Hood WB (1968) Regional venous drainage of the human heart. Brit Heart J 30: 105-109

Horiguchi M, Koizumi M, Isogai S (1988) Vv. bronchiales opening into atrium sinistrum. Acta Anat Nipponica 63: 384 (abstract)

Hutton WK (1915) An anomalous coronary sinus. J Anat Physiol 39: 407-413

International Anatomical Terminology (1998), Federative Committee on Anatomical Terminology (FCAT). Thieme, Stuttgart

Jacobs AK (1986) Coronary sinus interventions: clinical application. In: Mohl W, Faxon D, Wolner E (eds) Coronary sinus interventions - a new approach to interventional cardiology. Steinkopff Darmstadt, Springer New York, pp 27-39

Kennel AJ, Titus JL (1972) The vasculature of the human sinus node. Mayo Clin Proceed 47: 557-561

Kenner T, Moser M, Mohl W (1984) Wave reflection and pressure flow relations in the coronary circulation. In: Mohl W, Wolner E, Glogar D (eds) The coronary sinus. Steinkopff Darmstadt, Springer New York, pp 60-72

King A, McLelland J (1978) Anatomie der Vögel. Ulmer, Stuttgart

Kügelgen A v, Greinemann H (1958) Die Klappen in den menschlichen Nierenvenen, besonders an der Mündung der Nierenbeckenvenen. Z Zellforsch 47: 648-673

Lametschwandtner A, Mohl W (1984) The microcirculatory vascular bed of the dog's heart. A scanning electron microscopy study of vascular corrosion casts. In: Mohl W, Wolner E, Glogar D (eds) The coronary sinus. Steinkopff Darmstadt, Springer New York, pp 26-32

Lametschwandtner A, Lametschwandtner U, Weiger T (1990) Scanning electron microscopy of vascular corrosion casts - technique and applications: updated review. Scanning Microscopy 4: 889-941

Langer L (1880) Die Foramina Thebesii im Herzen des Menschen. Sitzungsber Math. Naturwiss. Classe, Kaiserl Akad d Wiss (Wien) 82 (Juniheft): 25-39

Langer L (1880) Über die Blutgefässe der Herzklappen des Menschen. Sitzungsber Math Naturwiss Classe, Kaiserl Akad d Wiss (Wien) 82 (Octoberheft):1-34

Langman J (1977) Medizinische Embryologie, 5th ed, Thieme, Stuttgart, pp 208-260

Lannelongue (1867) (see Tschabitscher 1984)

Lazar HL (1988) Coronary sinus interventions during cardiac surgery. Ann Thorac Surg 46: 475-482

Lechleuthner A, von Lüdinghausen M (1986) The functional architecture and clinical significance of the cardiac venous system with special reference to the venous valves and Thebesian veins. In: Mohl W, Faxon D, Wolner E (eds) Clinics of CSI. Springer, New York, pp 33-39

Lechleuthner A (1987) Das Venensystem des Säugetierherzens. Inaug Diss München, p 127

Lendrum B; Kondo B, Katz LN (1945) The role of Thebesian drainage in the dynamics of coronary flow. Amer J Physiol 143: 243-246

Leonhardt H (ed) (1987) Kreislaufsystem. In: Rauber-Kopsch Anatomie des Menschen, Bd 2. Thieme, Stuttgart, pp 30-61

Lewis FT (1904) The question of sinusoids. Anat Anz 25: 261-279

Lindeau KF, Romaniuk P (1983) Anatomie des Koronarsystems. In: Warnke H (ed) Chirurgie der koronaren Herzerkrankungen. Barth, Leipzig, pp 29-31

Lindsay FEF (1967) The cardiac veins of Gallus domesticus. J Anat 101: 555–568

Loop FD, Higgins TL, Panda R, Pearce G, Estafanous FG (1992) Myocardial protection during cardiac operations. J Thorac Cardiovasc Surg 104: 608–618

von Lüdinghausen M (1976) Pathologische myokardiale Perfusionsverteilung im Szintigramm und normales Koronarogramm. Dtsch Med Wschr 101: 1235 (Abstract)

von Lüdinghausen M, Ratajczyk-Pakalska E, Tschabitscher M, Maurer G, Glogar D, Mohl W (1984) Nomenclature: Venae cardiacae – cardiac veins. In: Mohl W, Wolner E, Glogar (eds) The coronary sinus. Steinkopff Darmstadt, Springer NewYork, pp 1–4

von Lüdinghausen M (1987) Clinical anatomy of the cardiac veins, Vv. cardiacae. Surg Radiol Anat 9: 159–168

von Lüdinghausen M, Lechleuthner A (1988) Atresia of the right atrial ostium of the coronary sinus. Acta Anat 131: 81–83

von Lüdinghausen M (1989) Aberrant course of the anterior interventricular part of the great cardiac vein in the human heart. Gegenbaur's Morphol Jahrb (Leipzig) 135: 475–478

von Lüdinghausen M, Schott C (1990) Microanatomy of the human coronary sinus and its major tributaries. In: Meerbaum S (ed) Myocardial perfusion, reperfusion, coronary venous retroperfusion. Steinkopff, Darmstadt, pp 93–122

von Lüdinghausen M, Ohmachi N, Boot C (1992) Myocardial coverage of the coronary sinus and related veins. Clin Anat 5: 1–15

von Lüdinghausen M, Ohmachi N, Chiba S (1994) The venous drainage of the myocardium in the human heart. In: Mohl W (ed) Coronary sinus interventions in cardiac surgery, Medical Intelligence Unit; Landes Bioscience, Georgetown, Texas, pp 11–26

von Lüdinghausen M, Ohmachi N, Besch S, Mettenleiter A (1995) Atrial veins of the human heart. Clin Anat 8: 169–189

von Lüdinghausen M, Ohmachi N, Chiba S (2000) The venous drainage of the myocardium of the human heart. In: Mohl W (ed) Coronary sinus interventions in cardiac surgery, 2nd edn, Medical Intelligence Unit 19, Landes Bioscience, Georgetown, Texas, pp 35–54

von Lüdinghausen M (2002) The clinical anatomy of the coronary arteries. Adv Anat Embryol Cell Biol (in press)

Lunkenheimer PP, Merker HJ (1973) Morphologische Studien zur funktionellen Anatomie der "Sinusoide" im Myokard. Z Anat Entwickl Gesch 142: 65–90

Lunkenheimer PP, Merker HJ (1974) Morphologie und Funktion eines intramyokardialen sinusoidalen Strömungsnetzes. Thoraxchir 22: 26–35

Lunkenheimer A, Merker HJ, Lunkenheimer PP (1984) Functional anatomy of the coronary sinusoids. In: Mohl W, Wolner E, Glogar D (eds) The coronary sinus. Steinkopff Darmstadt, Springer New York, pp 53–59

Malhotra VK, Tewari SP, Tewari PS, Agarwal SK (1980) Coronary sinus and its tributaries. Anat Anz 148: 331–332

Mantini E, Grondin CM, Lillehei CW, Edwards JE (1966) Congenital anomalies involving the coronary sinus. Circulation 33: 317–327

Marchand P, Gilroy JC, Wilson VH (1950) An anatomical study of the bronchial vascular system and its variations in disease. Thorax 5: 207–221

Maric I, Bobinac D, Ostojic L, Petkovic M, Dujmovic M (1996) Tributaries of the human and canine coronary sinus. Acta Anat 156: 61–69

Maros TN, Racz L, Plugor S, Maros TG (1983) Contributions to the morphology of the human coronary sinus. Anat Anz 154: 133–144

McAlpine WA (1975) Heart and coronary arteries. Springer, Berlin, Heidelberg, New York, pp 179–209

McMichael J, Mounsey JPD (1951) A complication following coronary sinus and cardiac vein catherisation in man. British Heart J 13: 397–402

Mechanik N (1934) Das Venensystem der Herzwände. Z Anat EntwGesch 103: 813–843

Meerbaum S (1984) The Beck era: a springboard for renewed research of coronary venous retroperfusion aimed at the treatment of myocardial ischemia. In: Mohl W, Wolner E, Glogar D (eds) The coronary sinus. Steinkopff Darmstadt, Springer New York, pp 320–327

Meerbaum S (2000) Coronary venous interventions. In: Mohl W (ed) Coronary sinus interventions in cardiac surgery, 2nd edn, Medical Intelligence Unit 19; Landes Bioschience, Georgetown Texas, pp 140–171

Menasche P, Kural S, Fauchet M, Lavergne A, Commin P, Bercot M, Touchot B, Georgiopoulos G, Piwnica A (1982) Retrograde coronary sinus perfusion: a safe alternative for ensuring cardioplegic delivery in aortic valve surgery. Ann Thorac Surg 34: 647-658

Mettenleiter A (2001) Adam Christian Thebesius (1686-1732) und die Entdeckung der Vasa Cordis Minima. Franz Steiner, Stuttgart

Mierzwa J, Kozielec T (1975) Variations of the anterior cardiac veins and their orifices in the right atrium in man. Folia Morphol (Warsz) 34: 125-132

Mochizuki S (1933) Vv. cordis. In: B Adachi (ed) Das Venensystem der Japaner. Kenkyusha, Tokyo, pp 41-64

Mohl W (1984a) The development and rationale of pressure-controlled intermittent coronary sinus occlusion. Wiener Klin Wschr 96: 20-25

Mohl W (1984b) Pressure-controlled intermittent coronary sinus occlusion. In: Mohl W, Wolner E, Glogar D (eds) The coronary sinus. Steinkopff Darmstadt, Springer, New York, pp 418-423

Mohl W, Neumann F, von Lüdinghausen M, Schreiner W, Simon P (1992) Cardioplegia for Coronary revascularisation in the presence of aortic regurgitation. In: Engelman RM, Levitsky S (eds) A textbook of cardioplegia for difficult clinical problems. Mount Kisco, NY, Futura publishing Company, pp 17-31

Mohl W (2000) Surgical coronary sinus interventions for myocardial protection. In: Mohl W (ed) Coronary sinus interventions in cardiac surgery, 2nd edn Landes Bioscience, Georgetown, Texas, pp 2-8

Moir TW, Eckstein RW, Driscol TE (1963) Thebesian drainage of the septal artery. Circ Res 12: 212-219

Moore KL (1985) Clinically oriented anatomy. 2nd edn, Williams & Wilkins, Baltimore, London, pp 97-133

Moore KL (1988) The developing human. 4th edn, Saunders, Philadelphia, pp 286-333

Moscovici M (1985) Luminal arteries in the human heart. XII International Anatomical Congress, London, August 11-17, (abstract)

Navaratnam V (1975) The human heart and circulation. Academic Press, London, pp 98-105

Nerantzis C, Antonakis E, Avgoustakis D (1978) A new corrosion casting technique. Anat Rec 191: 321-325

Netter FH (1976) Herz. Thieme, Stuttgart. p 16

Nguyen H, Doutriaux M, Leroy JP, Thuan RH (1975) Small veins of the heart auricle. Bull Assoc Anat (Nancy) 59: 955-967

Nguyen H, Nguyen M, Doutriaux M (1981) Atrioventricular or coronary sulcus (sulcus coronarius). Anat Clin 2: 329-341

Nomina Anatomica (1980) 5th edn, Williams & Wilkins, Baltimore, London

Nomina Anatomica (1989) 6th edn, International Anatomical Nomenclature Committee Churchill Livingston, Edinburgh

Nomina Anatomica, 8th edn, in H Feneis (1998) Pocket Atlas of Human Anatomy, ed W Dauber, Thieme, Stuttgart

Ono T, Shimohara Y, Okada K, Irino S (1986) Scanning electron microscopic studies on microvascular architecture of human coronary vessels by corrosion casts: normal and focal necrosis. Scanning Electron Microsc 1986/I: 263-270

O'Rahilly R (1971) The timing and sequence of events in human cardiogenesis. Acta anat 79: 70-75

Ortale JR, Marquez CQ (1998) Anatomy of the intramural venous sinuses of the right atrium and their tributaries. Surg Radiol Anat 20: 23-29

Ortale JR, Gabriel EA, Iost C, Marquez CQ (2001) The anatomy of the coronary sinus and its tributaries. Surg Radiol Anat 23: 15-21

Ovenfors CO (1956) Venous communications between the cardiac veins and the large venous trunks in the superior parts of the mediastinum. Radiology 46: 518-522

Pakalska E, Golab B (1980) Coronary circulation on the venous side in the human heart with the special references to the venae cordis minimae. In: Reinis Z, Pokorny J, Linhart J, Hild R, Schirger A (eds) Adaptability of vascular wall. Springer, Berlin, Heidelberg, New York, pp 679-681

Pakalska E, Fortak W, Golab B (1981) An occurrence of sphincter and regulator-like systems in the smallest cardiac veins of the human heart. Folia Morphol (Warsz) 29: 213-215

Parsonnet V (1953) The anatomy of the veins of the human heart with special reference to normal anastomotic channels. J Med Soc N J 50: 446-452

Peele TL (1932) A case of closed coronary sinus and left superior vena cava. Anat Rec 54: 83–86

Pejkovic B, Bogdanovic D (1992) The great cardiac vein. Surg Radiol Anat 14: 23–28

Pernkopf E (1937) Topographische Anatomie des Menschen. Vol 1 und 2. Urban & Schwarzenberg, Berlin, Wien, pp 360–361

Phillips SJ, Rosenberg A, Meir-Levi D, Pappas E (1979) Visualisation of the coronary microvascular bed by light and scanning electron microscopy and X-ray in the mammalian heart. Scanning Electron Microsc 111: 735–742

Piffer CR, Piffer MIS, Zorzetto NL (1990) Anatomic data of the human coronary sinus. Anat Anz 170: 21–29

Platzer W (1982) Atlas der topographischen Anatomie, Thieme, Stuttgart, pp 108–109

Potkin BN, Roberts WC (1987) Size of the coronary sinus at necropsy in subjects without cardiac disease and in patients with various cardiac conditions. Amer J Cardiol 60: 1418–1421

Pratt FH (1898) The nutrition of the heart through the vessels of Thebesius and the coronary veins. Amer J Physiol 1: 86–103

Prinzmetal M, Simkin B, Bergman HC, Kruger HE (1947) Studies on the coronary circulation. The collateral circulation of the normal human heart by coronary perfusion with radioactive erythrocytes and glass spheres. Amer Heart J 33: 420–442

Putz R, Pabst R (eds) (2000) Thorax. In: Sobotta Atlas der Anatomie des Menschen, Bd 2, 21st edn, Urban & Fischer München, Jena, pp 76–131

Ratajczyk-Pakalska E (1974) Studies on the cardiac veins in man and the domestic pig. Folia Morphol (Warsz) 33: 373–384

Ratajczyk-Pakalska E (1975) Arteriovenous anastomoses in the human myocardium. Folia Morphol (Warsz) 34: 285–292

Ratajczyk-Pakalska E (1977) Blood vessels supplying the left-ventricular cardiac muscle in man. Folia Morphol (Warsz) 36: 99–106

Ratajczyk-Pakalska E, Wagiel J, Kaminski M, Kolff WJ (1984) Automated image analysis for measurement of the area of the smallest cardiac veins in the ventricular myocardium. In: Mohl W, Wolner E, Glogar D (eds) The coronary sinus. Steinkopff Darmstadt; Springer New York, pp 33–39

Ratajczyk-Pakalska E and Kolff WJ (1984) Anatomical basis for the coronary venous outflow. In: Mohl W, Wolner E, Glogar D (eds) The coronary sinus. Steinkopff Darmstadt, Springer New York, pp 40–46

Ratajczyk-Pakalska E, Bloch P, Kulig A (1990) Angioarchitektonics of the venous vessel in the normal human myocardium. Folia Morphol (Warsz) 49: 26–33

Reed AF (1938/39) A left superior vena cava draining the blood from a closed coronary sinus. J Anat 73: 195–197

Rigby WFC, Graboys TB (1981) Current concepts and management of the preexcitation syndromes. J Cardiovasc Med 6: 277–293

Robb JS (1965) Comparative basic cardiology. Grune & Stratton New York, London, pp 123–140

Roberts JT (1958) Arteries, veins, and lymphatic vessels of the heart. In: Luisada AA (ed) Development and structure of the cardiovascular system. McGraw-Hill, New York, pp 85–118

Robinson K, Davies MJ, Krikler DM (1988) Type A Wolff-Parkinson-White syndrome obscured by left bundle branch block associated with a vascular malformation of the coronary sinus. Brit Heart J 60: 352–354

Rosen KM, Bauernfeind RA, Swiryn S, Dhingra RC, Wyndham CRC (1980) The significance of normal and anomalous atrioventricular conducting pathways in cardiac arrhythmias. Adv Intern Med 25: 277–302

Rosinia FA, Low FN (1986) Scanning electron microscopy of Thebesian ostia. Scanning Electron Microscopy IV: 1363–1369

Rychter Z, Ostadal B (1971) Mechanism of the development of coronary arteries in chick embryo. Folia Morph (Praha) 19: 113–124

Sallam IA, Kolff J (1973) A new surgical approach to myocardial revascularisation: Internal mammary to coronary vein anastomosis. Thorax 28: 613–616

Sarrazin R (1965) A propos des valvules du sinus coronaire. Arch Anat Path 13: 124–126

SchafflerGJ, Groell R, Peichel KH, Rienmüller R (2000) Imaging the coronary venous drainage system using electron-beam CT. Surg Radiol Anat 22: 35–39

Schaper W (1974) Zur Entstehung eines Kollateralkreislaufs bei Koronararterienverschlüssen. Dtsch Med Wschr 99: 2299-2302

Schaper W, Schaper J (1977) The coronary microcirculation. Am J Cardiol 40: 1008-1012

Scharf SM, Bromberger-Barnea B, Permutt S (1971) Distribution of coronary venous outflow. J Appl Physiol 30:657-662

Schippel K (1965) Über den mündungsnahen Abschnitt des Sinus coronarius cordis und die Valvula sinus coronarii. Anat Anz 117: 109-123

Schlant RC, Sonnenblick EH (1994) Normal physiology of the cardiovascular system. In: Schlant RC, Alexander RW (eds) Hurst's The heart, 8th edn, McGraw-Hill, New York, pp 113-151

Schneider J, Kappenberger L (1980) Das anatomische Substrat des Wolff-Parkinson-White Syndroms. Schweiz Med Wschr 110: 896-906

Schumacher B, Tebbenjohanns J, Pfeiffer D, Omran H, Jung W, Lüderitz B (1995) Prospective study of retrograde coronary venography in patients with posteroseptal and left-sided accessory atrioventricular pathways. Amer Heart J 130: 1031-1039

Schütz H (1914) Einige Fälle von Entwicklungsanomalie der Vena cava superior. Persistenz des linken Ductus Cuvieri. Virchows Arch Path Anat 216: 35-45

Sealy WC, Mikat EM (1983) Anatomical problems with identification and interruption of posterior septal Kent bundles. Ann Thorac Surg 36: 584-595

Shaner RF (1961) The development of the bronchial veins, with special reference to anomalies of the pulmonary veins. Anat Rec 140: 159-165

Shiki K, Masuda M, Yonenaga K, Asou T, Tokunaga K (1986) Myocardial distribution of retrograde flow through the coronary sinus of the excised normal canine heart. Ann Thorac Surg 41: 265-271

Siding A (1896) Über den Abschluss des Sinus coronarius cordis gegen den rechten Vorhof. Anat Anz 12: 274-277

Silver MA, Rowley NE (1988) The functional anatomy of the human coronary sinus. Amer Heart J 115: 1080-1084

Singer H, Bayer W, Reither M, Hinüber G.v. (1973) Koronargefäßanomalien und persistierende Myokardsinusoide bei Pulmonalatresie mit intaktem Ventrikelseptum. Basic Res Cardiol 68: 153-176

Smith GT (1962) The anatomy of coronary circulation. Amer J Cardiol 9: 327-342

Spalteholz W (1934) Die Thebesischen Venen. Anat Anz 79: 177-224

Staubesand J, Rulfs W (1958) Die Klappen kleiner Venen. Z Anat Entw Gesch 120: 392-423

Steding G, Seidl W (1980) Contribution to the development of the heart. Part I: normal development. Thorac Cardiovasc Surg 28: 386-409

Steding G, Jinwen X, Seidl W, Männer J, Xia H (1990) Developmental aspects of the sinus valves and the sinus venosus septum of the right atrium in human embryos. Acta Embryol 181: 469-475

Sun Y, Arruda MS, Otomo K, Beckman KJ, Nakagawa H, Calame J, Po S, Spector P, Lustgarten D, Herring L, Lazzara RNR, Jackman WM (2002) Role of the coronary sinus myocardial coat in epicardial posteroseptal and left posterior accessory pathways. Circulation, in press

Tandler J (1913) Anatomie des Herzens. In: von Bardeleben K, Handbuch der Anatomie, 3.Bd, 1.Abtg, Fischer Jena, pp 235-238

Tandler J (ed) (1926) Das Gefäßsystem. In: Tandler Lehrbuch der systematischen Anatomie, 3. Bd, Vogel, Leipzig, pp 77-97

Terminologia Anatomica (1998) International Anatomical Terminology, Federative Committee on Anatomical Terminology, Thieme, Stuttgart, pp 78-79

Thebesius AC (1708) De circulo sanguinis in corde. Disputatio Medica Inauguralis, Lugduni Batavorum, apud Abrahamum Elzevier, pp 3-19

Theman TE, Crosby DR (1981) Coronary artery steal secondary to coronary arteriovenous fistula. Can J Surg 24: 231-286

Töndury G (1970) Angewandte und topographische Anatomie, 4. Aufl. Thieme, Stuttgart, pp 64-67

Trento A, Zuberbuhler JR, Anderson RH, Park SC, Siewers RD (1988) Divided right atrium (prominence of the Eustachian and Thebesian valves). J Thorac Cardiovasc Surg 96: 457-463

Truex RC, Schwartz MJ (1951) Venous system of the myocardium with special reference to the conduction system. Circulation 4: 881-889

Truex RC, Angulo AW (1952) Comparative study of the arterial and venous systems of the ventricular myocardium with special reference to the coronary sinus. Anat Rec 113: 467-491.

Tschabitscher M (1984) Anatomy of the coronary sinus. In: Mohl W, Wolner W, Glogar D (eds) The coronary sinus. Steinkopff Darmstadt, Springer New York, pp 8–25

Tschabitscher M (1986) The so-called silent zone of the coronary sinus. In: Mohl W, Faxon D, Wolner E (eds) Coronary sinus interventions, a new approach to interventional cardiology. Steinkopff Darmstadt, Springer, New York, pp 11–14

Tsujioka K, Tomonaga G, Ogasawara Y, Nakai M, Tadaoka S, Goto M, Kajiya F (1984) Origin of phasic coronary venous flow and the capacitance of intramyocardial coronary veins. In: Mohl W, Wolner E, Glogar (eds) The coronary sinus. Steinkopff Darmstadt, Springer New York, pp 100–105

Unger K (1938) Beitrag zur Kenntnis der Venae cordis minimae (Thebesii) des menschlichen Herzens. Z Anat Entw Gesch 108: 356–375

Vajda J, Tomscik, van Doorenmaalen WJ (1972) Connections between the venous system of the heart and the epicardiac lymphatic network. Acta Anat 83: 262–274

Vieussens (1706) (see Mettenleiter A 2001)

Vlodaver DP, Amplatz MH, Burchell MH, Edwards MB (1976) Coronary heart disease, clinical, angiographic, and pathologic profiles. Springer, New York, Heidelberg, New York, pp 1–20

Voboril Z, Schiebler TH (1969) Über die Entstehung der Gefäßversorgung des Rattenherzens. Z Anat Entw Gesch 129: 24–40

Voboril Z, Schiebler TH (1970) Über die Entstehung der Gefäßversorgung des Rattenherzens. Verh Anat Ges 64: 259–264

Waldmeier E (1928) Das Rehherz (Cervus capreolus). Gegenbaur's Morphol Jb (Leipzig) 59: 567–598

Waller BF, Schlant RC (1994) Anatomy of the heart. In: Schlant RC and Alexander RW (eds) Hurst's The Heart, 8th edn, McGraw-Hill, New York, pp 59–112

Wearn JT (1928) The role of the Thebesian vessels in the circulation of the heart. J Exper Med 47: 293–316

Wearn JT, Mettier SR, Klumpp TG, Zschiesche LJ (1933) The nature of the vascular communications between the coronary arteries and the chambers of the heart. Amer Heart J 9: 143–164

Wenger R, Zandanell E (1969) Ein ungewöhnlicher Fall von Aneurysma des Sinus coronarius. Z Kreislaufforsch 58: 676–681

Williams PL, Bannister LH, Berry MM, Collins P. Dyson M, Dussek JE, Ferguson MWJ (eds) (1995). In: Gray's Anatomy, 38th British edn, Churchill Livingston, London. pp 1472–1503

Wright RR, Anson BJ, Cleveland HC (1948) The vestigial valves and the interatrial foramen of the adult human heart. Anat Rec 100: 331–355

Yater WM (1929) Variations and anomalies of the venous valves of the right atrium of the human heart. Arch Pathol 7: 418–441

Yater WM (1936) The paradox of Chiari's network. Amer Heart J 11: 542–553

Subject Index